40 *over* 40

40 Things *Every Woman Over 40 Needs to Know* About Getting Dressed

by Brenda Kinsel

Wildcat Canyon Press
A Division of Circulus Publishing Group, Inc.
Berkeley, California

Dedication

To my mother, Alma J. Reiten,
who made forty look like the prize

40 Over 40: 40 Things Every Woman Over 40 Needs to Know
about Getting Dressed
Copyright © 1999 by Brenda Kay Reiten Kinsel

Editorial Director: Roy M. Carlisle
Copyeditor: Jean Blomquist
Production Coordinator: Larissa Berry
Cover Design/Interior Design: Jenny M. Phillips of JuMP Studio
Illustrations: Jenny M. Phillips of JuMP Studio
Typesetting: Margaret Copeland
Typographic Specifications: Body text set in Cochin 11/15.
Heads set in Nobel Regular 32/32.

Printed in Canada
Library of Congress Cataloging-in-Publication Data
Kinsel, Brenda, 1952–
    Forty over forty : forty things every woman over forty needs to
know about getting dressed/ by Brenda Kinsel.
        p. cm.
    ISBN 1-885171-42-0 (alk. paper)
    1. Clothing and dress. 2. Fashion. 3. Middle-aged women. I. Title.

TT507 .K56 2000
646'.34—dc21
                                                                99-0462686

Distributed to the trade by Publishers Group West
10 9 8 7 6 5 4 3 2 1

Contents

Acknowledgements

There have been countless sources of support and inspiration throughout the process of writing this book. I wish to acknowledge those people who were there watering this project in its seedling stage and the many more who came forth to bring it to full bloom.

To my dad, Donald S. Reiten, who when I asked his advice about what to do with this nagging desire to write, told me to leap toward my dream, even providing the roadmap for how it would look. Your faith in me is my most prized possession.

To my delightful children, Trevor, Erin, and Caitlin, who were there for their writing mom at precisely the right moments with flowers, love notes, chocolates, sushi, and great escapes to hear jazz. You are forever my light, my joy, my happiness, my love. Thank you.

To my brothers, Brent, Kirk, and Todd, my sister-in-law Wendalyn (Wendy), my sister-in-law (close enough to count) Toni Bernbaum, and my three sisters by personal adoption— Patiricia Clure (yours forever), Joan Owen (my Norwegian sister), and dear Louise Elerding (my sis) who provided support as only family can, tirelessly. Thank you.

Before a book proposal even gets mailed out, there's a riotous cheering squad that backs up every baby step. Their participation and support has been rock steady. I am so grateful to you. Loving thanks to Kim Connor Kuhn, Linda Scheibel, Carl and Marie Dern, Randi Merzon, Persia Matine, Debra Newsholme, Helena Chenn, Cat Prince, Lynn Sydney, Ellen Rankin, Coffee Shop Guy, Cheri Hoggan, Larry Buttons,

Richard Rubia, Linda Anderson, Cheryl Little, Mary Ann Rolston, Sandra Paulsen, Tim Badger, and my 7 @ 7 group—Kate Comings, Joanne Harwood, Nadine Narita, Christa Ortman, Joan Owen, and Rosemary Shorrock.

These words wouldn't have found a page at all if not for my writing buddy, Christie Nelson, the best writing tool I could ever hope for. You had energy and enthusiasm for every paragraph—through every rewrite. My deepest appreciation and love to you, my devoted writing friend and beautiful woman—inside and out.

Deep thanks to my team at Wildcat Canyon Press. To Roy M. Carlisle, a most insightful, sensitive, and generous editor for his just-right touch and to Julienne Bennett, my publisher, who created a smart, nurturing home for 40 Over 40 right from the start. Thanks to my copyeditor, Jean M. Blomquist, who gave the kindest attention to these ideas and words. Your work was fabulous.

To Jenny Phillips, my illustrator, who is only the most brilliant and talented person I know. Your collaboration on this project has been the most delightful marriage of words and art. It inspired me from the very beginning. I am forever grateful.

To the *Pacific Sun* newspaper—thank you, Linda Xiques, editor, for the opportunity to espouse my ideas on your pages over these last years.

To my colleagues and fellow members of the Association of Image Consultants International. Your fellowship means everything to me. Warm thanks to those of you I've gotten to know especially through board participation and convention programs. You constantly inspire me. Special thanks to Debra Newsholme, Helena Chenn, Louise Elerding, Cat Prince, Chris

Ward, Angie Michael, Elaine Stoltz, Coralyn Lundell, Judith Rasband, Ginger Burr, Jean Gaffney, Lucille Grant, Lynn Henderson, Dominique Isbecque, Connie Coffey, Linda Buckman, Lynn Sydney, Cille Emery, Brenda Diehl, Judith Shimer, Colleen Abrie, Marjory DeRoeck, Mitra Sharei, Karen Snow, Angie Congdon, Denise Larkin, Kathleen Bresnahan, Nathania Apple, Susan Schwartz, Sharon Chrisman, Diane Parente, Gwen Mazer, Carla Mathis, Catherine Schuller, Judith Graham, Mari Lyn Henry, Jean Patton, Karen Brunger, Carolyn Gustafson, Donna Fujii, Marion Gellatly, Nancy Elorduy, Lisa Cunningham, Keiko Couch, Evana Maggiore, Donna Cognac, Jon Michael, and in loving memory, Jane Segerstrom.

Special thanks to Therese Post, Lynne Whiteside, Barbara Boungard, Gloria Untermann, Felix Magalong, Mark Bradshaw, Peter Sichel, Mickey Bolen, Laura Cohen, Terri Rouse, and Kyoo Park at Saks Fifth Avenue and to Ann Sandhu, Camille Chamberlin, Tony Dear, Jana Yim-Sarcona, and Angie Pickett at Nordstrom. Thanks for your great service to me and my clients.

To my clients—how can I thank you? Your honesty and beauty illuminates every page of this book. Working with you is my deep privilege. Thank you so much.

To Sallie Welles—your counsel always makes me see everything in the best light. Thank you. To Sunny Yates and Gary Yates for their brilliant work in designing innovative and effective solutions. Sunny, you created the framework for ease and grace, fun and adventure—when I thought I'd run out of steam. I could *never* have done this without your brilliant coaching.

To my gardener, Robert Moore. Your landscape of flowers,

words, and ideas have been a haven for my senses and a great comfort to my heart throughout this process. Thank you for your wisdom and friendship.

To Paul Johnson—for your deep friendship, your tireless interest, your understanding of the creative process, your honest love—you are a beacon of light that shines brightly. Forever, thanks.

Editorial Notes

The names of many of the products mentioned in these pages are registered trademarks, belonging to their owners. We fully acknowledge the rights of these owners.

Some individuals' names have been changed and certain characteristics have been disguised to protect contributors' privacy.

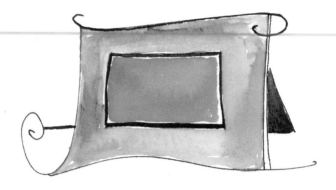

Introduction

MY MOTHER WAS FORTY the day the photographer came to our house on Cherry Court and lined us kids up behind my parents, who were sitting shoulder to shoulder on the piano bench. I've never forgotten how she looked. She was in her mint-green knit suit. Her brooch and earrings were the same gold tone as the buttons on her closed jacket. Her soft strawberry-blond hair was in tamed curls framing her bespeckled, confident face.

I was a teenager looking through a different lens that day, but what I captured was just as permanent an image as the portrait that hung for years on our dining room wall. While the photographer was setting up his tripod, I was looking into the future. In that moment, watching my mom settle onto the piano bench, I saw how profound it was to be a woman at forty. Forty meant freedom. When you were forty, you could be yourself, you didn't have to live up to other's expectations. Forty meant you could wear whatever you wanted to, because by then you were your full, radiant self, not a copy of someone else. I could hardly wait to be just like my mom, an original, in her mint-green suit on that fall day in North Dakota.

Now, twenty-some years later, it could be me sitting on that piano bench with my teenaged daughters and my son posing behind me. I've grown up. Not only am I in my forties myself, but it's also my good fortune to be working every day with women in their forties, dressing them to look their beautiful selves.

I wonder if it really was easier back then, or did my mom just make it look easy? Life seems so complicated today. Women have been crazy busy. Look around. We've climbed the corporate ladder, survived a divorce or two or three, been to therapy. If you're forty, you may have earned a black belt in juggling careers and family. I know you. While you're making time to mentor a coworker, you're also closely following the basketball or soccer seasons of your kids, consoling one friend through a breakup, or helping another one plan her wedding. Chances are you're the most likely one to be neglected. While you're chasing life down the fast lane, you're not sure how to dress yourself anymore. Your wardrobe's been slogging along in the slow lane for a decade or maybe two.

Where does a **real woman** go for relevant advice on style and clothes?

Fashion magazines? They're filled with pages of twenty-year-olds weighing less than a hundred pounds. Do you take the advice of your teenaged daughter—in orange hair and skimpy

T-shirt, with a pierced tongue and belly-button ring? No. When you manage to grab a minute to shop for yourself, what do you find on the racks? Retro fashions in Day-Glo colors, showing up again like a bad dream. Aaaugh! This is hard work! Everything's stopped making sense.

To confuse the issue even more, you're living in a different body. Your shape is changing, and your hair and attitudes are too. Where do you fit in? I've heard the lamenting. If you could make it all go away, you would. You may be older and wiser, but opening your closet door still brings you to your knees. You could have written the Roy Lichtenstein caption on the T-shirt that says, "I feel like such a failure! I've been shopping for over twenty years, and I still don't have anything to wear!" Should you just give up?

Hold everything! Amidst the world's clatter, it's time to do the unthinkable—to slow down, turn the focus on yourself, and do a major check-in. Who are you right now? Get current. Take a good long look, discover yourself anew. It's the right time to take a look in the mirror and make peace with this body, these arms, these thighs, these gorgeous lips, and this hair flecked with gray. This precious body of yours has made it through one million comparisons and has defied the look of the Kate Moss print ads on the sides of city buses.

It's time to invite a new love affair into your life—a love affair with your every line, every tooth, every toenail, every facial expression, every whim and desire. Passionate, wild, crazy, frivolous, impulsive—make it a love affair with yourself.

You've earned it. There are no more excuses. There's no time to waste, nothing's more important. You have collected half a lifetime of laughs, wisdom, accomplishments, mistakes, integrity, and experience. You've kept getting better and better. Now it's time to express that on the outside—confidently, boldly.

There is freedom at forty, the freedom I saw in my mother's eyes, in her sure smile. With a little excavating and renovating of attitudes, you'll be wearing that freedom too. It's under the surface, waiting to reveal itself. You'll find it in these forty chapters of fashion advice. You'll learn how to combine looks, passion, personality, and preferences into the perfect recipe for wearing clothes and accessories—while having delicious fun.

Forget about problem areas! Go somewhere else to hear about camouflage tricks. You'll be too busy falling in love with yourself when you put the focus on what works (a great smile, pretty skin, shapely calves). Other body parts will quiet down and assume their proper proportion. You'll find the correlation between your personality and preferences and discover how to wear them proudly. You'll learn how to shop for a bathing suit with dignity and courage, what to wear while going through a divorce, what to do instead of (or until) plastic surgery, and how to walk away from clothing with "potential" and only buy what works.

I won't ask you to do anything I haven't already done in my forties. I've been the mom who frantically shopped for school lunch ingredients at 7 A.M. in my accessorized jammies. Following my own advice on dressing for a high school reunion, I snagged a sweetheart at mine. I've given in to friends who insisted I'd lost ten pounds when all I'd really done was lift up my bra straps and loosen my belt. It's all doable. My clients in my style and wardrobe consulting business prove it to me every single day.

I invite you to zero in on the ordinary thing that you do everyday— getting dressed— and turn it into an opportunity for **personal expression, peace, and joy** *beyond words.*

After you've done your homework, it'll be so much easier to turn off the screaming consumer ads, ignore questionable advice from teenaged daughters or well-meaning friends, and trust yourself. You can and will love how you look in clothes. Come on, I'm going to show you how.

Your Clothes
Have Expired

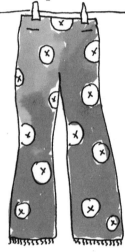

*It's better to learn to
say good-by early
than late . . .*

~JESSAMYN WEST,
LOVE, DEATH AND THE LADIES DRILL TEAM

IN THE LAST FIFTEEN YEARS, you have probably changed car models, magazine subscriptions, restaurants, doctors, hairdressers. Why? Because your taste has changed, your income has changed, your values have changed, *you've changed*. At forty, you're a lifetime or two from who you were at twenty-five. Your clothes need to change to reflect you, now, this decade, this year, this moment.

Think of clothes as perishables. Someone out there is dying to tell you that those acid-wash jeans with the zippers at the ankles should have been disposed of in '86. Now if the fashion industry just worked like the food industry, this would be a piece of cake.

Remember the old days, before expiration dates were

stamped on foods? You'd go to clean out the refrigerator and there was no telling what you'd find under the lid of the tub of cream cheese. But now, thanks to the brilliant vice president of some company like Land-O-Lakes, your daughter can ask while standing with the fridge door open, "Hey, Mom, has the cream cheese gone bad?" And all you do is say, "I don't know. What's the date on the bottom?"

"July 19th."

And if it's October, it's easy. You say, *"Throw it out, honey."* With expiration dates on food, there's no more lifting lids to see if what's inside has grown a fur coat or turned colors like mood rings. All we do is tip the container upside down, read the date stamped on the bottom, and then toss it out with barely a flush of guilt.

If only it could be as easy to recognize clothes that have gone bad.

Clothes hang around for decades. If they were food, they'd have escalated to advanced science experiments like those you find in cereal bowls under your teenagers' beds. Smooth silks would become corduroys, solid greens would turn into madras plaids. Dehydration would make dresses shrivel up three sizes.

If clothes were like food, it would be easy to throw them out once they'd passed their expiration date. You wouldn't need a second opinion about the floral dress with the three-inch-high puff sleeves or the '80s football-shoulder-padded anythings. You'd dispose of them, maybe even in the same trash can that the cream cheese went in.

But no, people have so many hang-ups about letting go of clothes! You don't have to convince me. I can see it with my own eyes. Those acid-wash jeans with the zippers at the ankles are still in great shape. They have no rips, no tears, no stains. You haven't worn them in eight years, but maybe they'll come back, you protest. If we're lucky, they won't.

No matter what, most old clothes don't get better with age, they just get antiquated. And those leftover clothes worn today only make you look older and dated. That's a grave disservice to you. You've grown up! You've gotten smarter, cuter, more clever. Don't let those old clothes drag you down, spreading rumors about you that aren't true.

If you don't like hearing it from me, take this test. The quickest way to find out if your clothes have expired is to take a couple of items in question to a consignment store. When the owner hands back your acid-wash jeans and you protest with her like you did with me — "But they are in great condition! Someone could get a lot of wear out of these!" — what the store owner is thinking but is too nice to say is, "Lady, that was last decade. We can't give these things away. Get over it."

The hard truth is that those savvy shoppers who peruse consignment stores aren't going to want your dinosaurs. Just like you don't want theirs. Those consignment store owners are smart. They know old from new, style from crap. They won't accept your duds unless they think someone else will like them enough to buy them. Don't be a pest. They know their customers better than you do.

You could give your jeans to your sister or your friends, but that requires face-to-face contact and you can't pout if they look at you funny and say no, thanks. If guilt runs in your family, you can always give a relative your rejects, which they'll pass on to the next relative after they've stored them in their garage for six months.

One group that might get a kick out of your vintage duds is your teenaged daughters and their friends. If you're hanging onto clothes because you think particular styles will come back again, you're half right. Styles do get recycled—in new fabrics, with new details. If you have items from another era in your closet, give them to the kids and go out and buy the new version. Twenty-year-old clothing is not youthful on older women, but it can be charming on the young. You'll be the neighborhood hero for a day. Hopefully they'll clean you out of your moldy oldies.

The thing about expired clothes is that everyone else can see it so much faster than you can. When you've been living with something for long, you tend to make a gazillion excuses for it if you're not wearing it. You're blind to the details of this staggeringly bad garment—the epaulets, the oversized patch pockets. Like the stain on the couch, it's obvious to others, but you're used to it and don't see it anymore.

That's why we need expiration dates sewn inside clothing. Flashy, trendy, bright-colored clothes would have a six-month usage date. You'd find it on a tag sewn along the side seam, next to the care instructions. It would say "Better If Used By 19 December 00." Neutral colors and simple, classically detailed clothing would be less perishable. "Better If Used By 22 June 02."

You would stop consuming all that energy dragging an unsellable item from consignment store to consignment store, relative to relative. Maybe in the middle of the night, on trash night, you decide to toss the damn thing away with the expired cream cheese. If Richard, your night-owl neighbor, catches you at the curb and asks you, "Why are you throwing away those perfectly good pants?" you could just reassure him. You'd point to the inside tag. "See? See here? It says '17 September 95.' It's expired, Richard!"

But until then, it's time to face the truth that those clothes have expired, tag or no. **Get them out of sight, out of the house, out of your mind**—even if it makes you feel insecure. The immense mental energy that it takes to sustain an expired wardrobe can be released into much more productive and pleasurable activities—like learning how to dress your deli-cious *current* self.

Bless those expired beauties. They served you well. They can be passed on to others through charities such as Goodwill where they will serve someone else. Time for you to move on.

The "M" Word

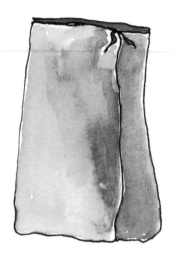

Don't compromise yourself.
You are all you've got.

~JANIS JOPLIN, QUOTED IN
READER'S DIGEST, APRIL 1973

2

I STUMBLED UPON THIS quite by accident—a word that could scare the spit out of a woman in her forties. It's not a swear word, it's not a dirty word, but it's so offensive that if you say it to a forty-year-old, she shivers like she has cooties all over her. What is it about the word "matronly" that makes a woman ill? I checked my dictionary for clarification. Here's what the *American Heritage Dictionary* says about the "M" word: **"matronly**: A married woman or a widow especially a mother of dignity, mature age, and established social position." Now that doesn't sound bad, does it? But I know you'd agree— no one in our age group wants that word anywhere near her.

When I think of "matronly," Esther Anderson comes immediately to mind. Her husband ran the grocery store and the post office where I grew up. In a town of seventy-five people, he was a well-respected man. When he died of a sudden heart attack, Esther was a prominent widow in town. I wasn't ten years old, but I remember how she looked. She wore dull-colored housedresses in tiny floral prints, thick opaque looking nylons that kept wanting to curl down to her stout ankles. Her undergarments couldn't contain her full bosom, which chose to rest at her waist. Her slip hung lower than her dress in the back. She had a musical voice that never went flat even after her loving Roy died. She held her chin up high, her gray hair flattened close to her head with bobby pins. Esther was matronly. She was in her mid-forties. She was old. I admired her strength but never thought to walk in her fashion footsteps.

Left on our own, without the aid of a dictionary this time, we can come up with our own synonyms for matronly—dowdy, dumpy, out-of-date. Not generally the coveted look for a woman still breathing.

At forty-something, you may be in a matronly rut yourself. Maybe you're not particularly dignified and your established social position is that of the person who sits in the corner chair at the coffee shop every morning. You're not married or widowed so you don't qualify to be matronly, but you fear that you somehow have the look. Mostly it's a look characterized by neglect. A woman has fallen into a rut and has little hope of getting out of it.

I know from experience that if I want to steer someone away from a bad choice, after I've tried reason and fact—"I know you're very fond of the earth, but mud brown just isn't your color" or "I know you've worn earrings the size of fried eggs for ten years, but really, we moved past that look twenty years ago"—there's always the "M" word. It works much like a cattle prod on a straying cow. It gets a woman to move quickly, to leap off the cliff with no regrets, to suddenly find religion. I choose my words carefully, and in that musical voice that I remember from Esther Anderson I say, "It just makes you look so . . . matronly."

Here are some items that have the "M" word written all over them.

The #1 most matronly clothing item on the planet is the stiff, long A-line denim skirt, especially with pleats. Make no excuses for this clothing item. Treat it like typhoid fever. Get it out of your closet immediately. In any form, on any body, it is *matronly.*

Decorated sweatshirts with matching pull-on pants is a great idea for toddlers but not for grown women. If this is a habit you're in, you've got to get yourself out of it. Sweats are the updated housedress. Wearing them once in a while is one thing, but generally the message of this ensemble is "I'm not doing anything with my life anymore. Don't expect me to finish a complete sentence."

Bare feet in high heels with jeans are more dated than Wilt Chamberlain. And while we're on the subject of jeans, black sheer hose or any sheer hose with jeans say "old lady." Jeans are a casual, coarse, rough fabric. Wearing nylons with them is like wearing running shoes with an evening gown. Instead wear a thin sock inside a non-dressy shoe with a sturdy heel or wear a boot.

Wearing bras where your boobs are spilling out over the cup and the surplus jiggles when you walk is matronly. Upgrade your underwear. You need a new bra, one with a full cup. Demi-cups are not for you. Go to a lingerie department where a foundation person will measure and fit you with the right undergarments.

Bad fit is matronly. Have your clothes altered so hemlines hang evenly. Don't wear clothes too tight.

Promise me you'll clean up your bad habits and kick your wardrobe into rehab. Don't come out until you've thrown out the denim skirt, you've vowed to do away with the heels and jeans, and you've curtailed the jiggling. I mean it.

Don't make me use the "M" word.

Organize Your Closet and Have More Time for Sex

I've got to relearn what I was supposed to have learned.

~Sylvia Ashton-Warner, *Myself*

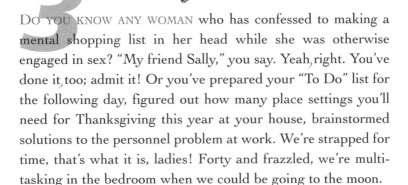

DO YOU KNOW ANY WOMAN who has confessed to making a mental shopping list in her head while she was otherwise engaged in sex? "My friend Sally," you say. Yeah, right. You've done it, too; admit it! Or you've prepared your "To Do" list for the following day, figured out how many place settings you'll need for Thanksgiving this year at your house, brainstormed solutions to the personnel problem at work. We're strapped for time, that's what it is, ladies! Forty and frazzled, we're multi-tasking in the bedroom when we could be going to the moon.

With all the practice we've had, sex is best after forty and damn if I'm not determined to find you an extra hour a day so you can enjoy every step of your stairway to heaven.

I've studied each and every one of the twenty-four hours in

a day, and I've located a time waster and energy sapper. It's called "Closet Morass." Let my pals Cheryl and Nancy provide you with the visual aids.

Cheryl B., forty-seven and a software designer, opens her closet doors at 6:15 A.M. and views everything she's ever owned since high school. It takes nearly an hour to weed through the smooshed pleated skirts, fringed jackets, and cheerleading outfits to find something appropriate to go to work in. After someone looks at her funny at work, she wonders if she got it right.

Nancy P, forty-three, is a focused and confident career counselor. But in her own closet she suffers anxiety attacks. Belts snake out of a ragged shopping bag in a dark corner. Teetering out of reach on a high shelf is a shoebox full of scarves with stunning potential but which threaten to inbreed with the photos spilling out of a torn box nearby. Nancy desperately wants to look pulled together. Skirts call out to her, but something's wrong with each one. The black one needs hemming, the taupe one is too small—still. Now she feels guilty and mad at herself and soon nothing looks good. After forty-five minutes of closet analysis, she succumbs to wearing the same gray pants, white blouse, and yellow cardigan sweater that she wears every day. She leaves for work—defeated, uninspired, grumpy.

I have a plan to eliminate getting bummed out in the mornings and to experience nothing but bliss instead. Just think of being able to open your closet doors and see everything inside. All the clothes in front of you look fabulous on you and work 100 percent, right now, just as they are. Getting dressed would take you five minutes and you'd feel great about yourself, leaving roughly fifty-five carefree minutes to focus on other things.

How could you ever get your closet—and clothes—to work like this? I will it down for you.

Step one: Block out an afternoon. Turn off the phone and the TV. Put on some Celine Dion, Patsy Kline, or Aretha Franklin. Crank it up loud, baby. Roll up your sleeves, open up that closet door and regardless of what's staring back at you, keep your eye on the prize—that extra hour in the morning.

Step two: Your closet is your personal shrine to the art of getting dressed and should hold only clothing and accessories. Banish the old living room drapes stuffed in the back, the stack of high school yearbooks, the pool sticks, the boxes of pictures that have been waiting to go into photo albums for years, plus whatever you think you're hiding from the kids. Don't you know that's the first place they look? Out, out, all of it, *out.* You store spices in your spice rack, your car in the garage, your toilet paper in the bathroom. You store clothes in your closet and accessories in or near your closet.

Step three: Hey, if you're going to have sex, have wonderful sex, okay? Not so-so sex. Same with clothes hanging in your closet. Take a look at every single item in there and keep only those clothes that are wonderful—ditch the rest. You're phenomenal! You're incredible! There's not a close second anywhere to your fabulous self. So don't hang onto anything that brings you down, that's "okay" but not "great." Come on! Stay with me. Don't make excuses for an outfit bought on sale that didn't quite fit and still doesn't; the well-meaning gifts from relatives who know your name but not your style; the twenty-five ragged T-shirts that you might put on if you ever wash your car by hand. What remains between those walls fits you *now* looks great, and vies like your best friends for your attention: "Wear me next time! Wear me!"

Step four: While you've been inspecting the troops in there, set aside all items needing attention—buttons that need reinforcing, hemlines that need to be secured again, a skirt that needs taking in or out. And make a plan to have those things taken care of within two weeks. Put it on your calendar. Don't tell me you'll do it later. It's that dropped detail that will pop into your mind in your next love lock.

Step five: Buy a beautiful box and call it your souvenir box. Put clothing and jewelry in it that you love dearly but will never wear again—the macaroni necklace Johnny made in second grade for you on Mother's Day, your favorite pants that split at the knees when you were roller skating in Golden Gate Park, the Guatemalan huipils you wore in the '70s. They're gems, absolutely, but they don't belong in your working wardrobe.

How are you doing so far? You're halfway there. Take a five-minute break and indulge in a fantasy, then get back to work.

Step six: Recycle your wire hangers. Buy plastic tubular hangers in one color or clear plastic hangers, or wooden ones. Hang all your clothes in the same direction on your hanger of choice. Good hangers protect your clothing and give them staying power.

Step seven: Arrange everything in your closet by color from dark to light. All black items together, then brown, reds, blues, ivory, then white. Opening your closet to colors grouped together is like opening a new box of sixty-four Crayola crayons. The colors are all lined up—blue-violet next to violet, then red-violet. Besides being gorgeous and soothing on the eyes, this arrangement lets you be more creative and playful, pairing items together that were mere acquaintances in the past.

Step eight: Arrange your accessories so they are visible. Scarves hang in holders on one end of your clothes rack. Belts and necklaces hang on tie racks. Keep your jewelry in baskets on a shelf in the closet or on top of a bureau. Line up your shoes under your clothes, dark to light.

Now your closet is orderly. Like a Zen garden, it looks tended and cared for. See all those clothes hanging in there by color? They're all your favorites, no bad apples in the bunch, so choosing something to wear is easy.

Tonight when you go to bed, your mind is at rest, knowing that the morning light will come through those windows and you'll open your closet door, choose something glorious to celebrate the day in, walk out, and shine.

It will have taken you five minutes to get dressed, the kids will have left for school. Neither you nor your honey has to be at work until nine—so, go ahead, get undressed. (Remember: it will only take five minutes to get dressed again!) Get under the covers with your sweetie and watch fifty-five minutes of *An Affair to Remember* on your VCR,

unless you can think of
something **else** to do…

Update Your Attitude

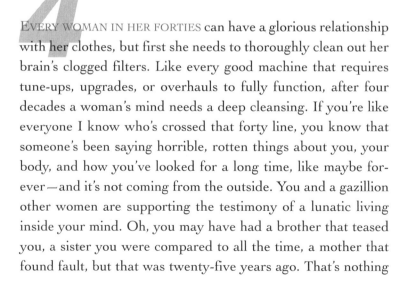

*There is no excellent beauty
that hath not some strangeness
in the proportion.*

~Francis Bacon, "Of Beauty"

4 Every woman in her forties can have a glorious relationship with her clothes, but first she needs to thoroughly clean out her brain's clogged filters. Like every good machine that requires tune-ups, upgrades, or overhauls to fully function, after four decades a woman's mind needs a deep cleansing. If you're like everyone I know who's crossed that forty line, you know that someone's been saying horrible, rotten things about you, your body, and how you've looked for a long time, like maybe forever—and it's not coming from the outside. You and a gazillion other women are supporting the testimony of a lunatic living inside your mind. Oh, you may have had a brother that teased you, a sister you were compared to all the time, a mother that found fault, but that was twenty-five years ago. That's nothing compared to the self-inflicted wounding that women do to themselves nearly unconsciously. I bet if someone recorded the crap that flies around inside a woman's head and amplified it in a shopping mall, the place would be deserted in five minutes. It's disgusting, degrading, horrifying to listen to. No one wants to be around that constant needling, the ruthless and defeating habit of comparing yourself to others or to who you were twenty years ago when you were blonder, thinner, smoother. It's a critical nagging that runs on a loop tape like your incoming phone message, repeating itself constantly, "I don't like my legs. My right eye droops funny. My arms are too flabby." From the texture of the hair on top of your head to the feet that keep you upright, you can find fault with much of your body and can spout off a rapid-fire, rote litany of imagined "problem areas." It's a nasty habit. Those critical barbs stick to brain matter like barnacles to rock and keep us from our joy.

Here's what I want you to do. Cut it out! Stop. Finis. That's it. Declare it's over, kaput, finished. I want you to take that critical, mean-spirited, one-sided conversationalist and talk back to it out loud or write it a good-bye letter: "Thank you for sharing, now come sit here, and be quiet." Tuck that big know-it-all under your arm, announce that there's someone new in charge and that it has been relinquished from its duties. Believe me, that beast will be relieved. He or she has had it, too, and is ready to turn right around and fill in what's been missing—the glorious appreciation for who you are, inside and out.

Angeles Arrien, Ph.D., in her book *The Four-Fold Way*, talks about the addictive pattern of being fixated on what's not working rather than on what is. She says, "When this addiction is fully disengaged, we begin to look at the blessings, gifts, talents

and resources that are available to us in our lives."
**Instead of focusing on fault, I implore
you to leave the past behind and
look at yourself in a fresh way—
through the eyes of a generous, kind,
and passionate lover, eagerly discovering
every nuance of your body, mind,
and spirit, *enjoying the perfection
of your humanness*, responding
enthusiastically to every part of you
that is revealed. Let your love penetrate
and warm those fierce, old judgments
until they dissolve away.**

You know how to do this, you've done it over and over with others. You've met a man. At first glance, his eyebrows seem to be crashing into his eyes, you notice his skin is rough and worn, probably by the sun and the sea. His smile is loose and crooked. As your fondness for him grows, the rough skin and the awkward features all soften and meld into this delicious package. His beauty is unique, as is yours, ready to be discovered and appreciated. It's been there all along. You just haven't been tracking it.

There is no time to hesitate. This is an urgent matter. Clean out that sharp-tongued filter in your brain. Start relaying gorgeous messages to yourself now that you've tamed that beast who used to live inside you. Throw the damn bathroom scale out the window. Get rid of the calendar you recorded your weight on. Get caught up with yourself. Connect to who you are right now, this minute. Touch that sweet gorgeous body of yours. Get naked and look at every angle of it in a full-length mirror. Appreciate ten things about your body right now—like how, without any direction from you at all, your eyeballs stay moist, or how without being poked or prodded, your skin stays stretched over every bone and muscle, protecting the machinery that tirelessly keeps functioning while you're busy doing other things. Or notice how your body automatically has a smile ready in case you need one, your laughter stored in your belly, ready at any moment to rise and be pushed out by your lungs, even as your heart stands alert to feel the sorrow at your friend's mother's imminent death. This is your precious body, your clever mind, your generous spirit. Now is the time to celebrate their existence, usefulness, and beauty.

I am in front of bodies all the time—bodies that fit in clothes from size 0 to size 26—and I've witnessed this "wonderment" with nearly every client when she sees herself anew. I've commented on a forty-eight-year-old woman's great broad shoulders and pointed out what terrific proportion those shoulders are to her hips. She confesses that all her life she's been self-conscious because she thought her shoulders were "too big." Another brilliant client in her late forties questions the V-neck shell I've put on her in a dressing room. "But I didn't think I could wear that," she says. "Shouldn't I be covering up my neck and upper chest?" she wondered. And all the while, I am staring at a beautiful neck and upper chest, which she should enjoy fully.

Remember that there is no one recipe for beauty; it is expressed in countless ways. In nature, everything does its best to be all that it can be. A rose doesn't beg to be like a lily. A rose exudes "rose-ness." A tulip masters being a tulip. A hyacinth grows up to be a glorious hyacinth. Whatever your color, scent, texture, shape, design—express it as fully as a rose, tulip, or hyacinth.

What you've been thinking are your flaws could very well be your strongest assets. Fall in love with your full face, crooked nose, short fingers. Honor your distinctiveness. Stand tall, square your shoulders, walk proud. Dust off the words of your doting aunt who said, "Don't try to be a xeroxed copy of someone else, honey. You're the original."

Clothes will help you express your originality, the beautiful woman that you have grown into. So finish that upgrade on your mind. Practice every day to clean out that mental filter. With a new attitude, clothes are about to become a new devoted friend to your body, mind, and soul.

Reasons to Get Dressed

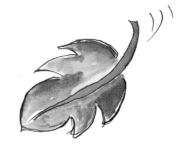

The first thing the first couple did after committing the first sin was to get dressed. Thus Adam and Eve started the world of fashion, and styles have been changing ever since.

~"GILDING THE LILY," *TIME* (NOVEMBER 8, 1963)

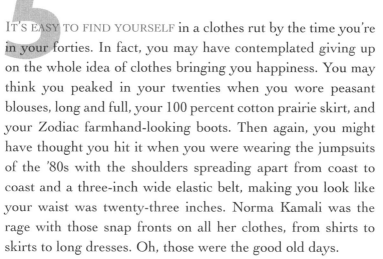

IT'S EASY TO FIND YOURSELF in a clothes rut by the time you're in your forties. In fact, you may have contemplated giving up on the whole idea of clothes bringing you happiness. You may think you peaked in your twenties when you wore peasant blouses, long and full, your 100 percent cotton prairie skirt, and your Zodiac farmhand-looking boots. Then again, you might have thought you hit it when you were wearing the jumpsuits of the '80s with the shoulders spreading apart from coast to coast and a three-inch wide elastic belt, making you look like your waist was twenty-three inches. Norma Kamali was the rage with those snap fronts on all her clothes, from shirts to skirts to long dresses. Oh, those were the good old days.

You could have been someone who was clothes cocky for

years. You fearlessly got away with just about anything. Then one day you wake up and the jig is up. Everything makes you look goofball. Your confidence slips away like runs in panty-hose—*fast*. You look at young people and think their clothes are bizarre. You're not comfortable in their camp. At the last minute, otherwise brilliant women shopping for an event find themselves disgusted with the clothes, disgusted with them-selves, disgusted that after all these years, shopping has become a bitch. Clothes really look like the problem.

Maybe you've relied on a certain sales clerk to help you out. Then she moves to another store, and another. You follow her around town and end up with mismatched clothes jammed in your closet without a plan. Or vendors you counted on are letting you down. Your favorite lines of clothes went out of business when retail dried up in the '80s. Or the designers keep switching influences and you're not tracking with them. After a couple of seasons, it's easy to feel lost.

Stop right there, forty-ish young woman; you're not going to slip down that slope of resignation. You've got so many more things in your favor now that you're forty. You need to capitalize on your good fortune.

There's every reason to dress well now. At twenty you didn't know anything. At thirty you were obsessively striving to reach the stars. At forty you're at the top of your game. You still have youth on your side, you're healthy, you're comfortable with your sexuality, you have perspective.

Clothes are a lot more than things you throw on to keep from getting cold or getting arrested. Wearing flattering colors can make up for lack of sleep. The right proportions of a suit can knock years and pounds off your driver's license. A column of color in smooth fabrics can appear to increase your IQ. A pleasing, appropriate ensemble can get you a promotion, a date, win your case, give you instant confidence, comfort, and personal pleasure.

Clothes *celebrate, announce, advertise,* and *declare yourself.* You hardly have a more

powerful tool for life.

What's the strongest position you can take at forty? It's to educate yourself about yourself. Perhaps for the first time. Before you buy any new clothes, I want you to go to school. Start with chapters 7, 8, 9, and 10 in this book. I'm going to give you exercises to do. You'll discover your **own style recipe**. Stores provide you a menu with their racks of clothes and you'll look at the menu and select your choices confidently. It's that easy.

You'll want the results that doing your homework will provide. Clothes are expressive and entertaining. Besides protecting you from the elements, the right clothes have the uncanny ability to make you feel at ease, more beautiful, more assured, more "yourself" than you feel with no clothes on at all.

Need more reasons for consciously getting dressed in your fourth decade? Seeing someone "put together" is a gift, a tiny miracle, a beauty burst—like a rose bush in bloom, a babbling brook, a perfectly baked chocolate chip cookie. It's delicious. You've found yourself waiting on a park bench, in an office, or at a concert and watched people go by. You've admired the harmony of a woman who is well-dressed, demonstrating her personal style. She looks like herself. That brief moment of appreciation can alter your mood, make you feel good. You can be that gift to your family, your friends, your coworkers, even strangers on the street. Everyone lives longer and better with beauty in their lives.

How about this one? Getting dressed may be the sexiest act you perform all day. And, like sex, it can be different every time. You dress every day. Why not take advantage of this creative experience and indulge yourself in the sensuality of color, texture, pattern, and drape of a fabric? When you've combined pleasing elements—a cuddly sweater in a favorite color, your grandmother's pearls (which remind you of her ruby-red rouged cheeks), pants that drape languidly on you—you look great, and then you feel great, and, big surprise, life also turns out great that day.

Here's the thing. When you're in clothes that bring out your essence, your uniqueness, everyone sees *you*—you, not necessarily your clothes. It's like the world is looking at you with 20/20 vision. And better yet, you can see yourself more clearly. Your outer appearance can validate and mirror your interior. Clothes help remind you of who you are. "Hey, I'm a sophisticated person! I'm smart, experienced. I'm funny." Clothes help do the talking.

You've got forty years or more under your belt. You're old enough to figure out what works, what doesn't, and to admit that you want to know the difference.

You know what you love, what you hate. You're old enough to choose to do the right thing, especially when it's for your own good, even though making changes may be uncomfortable. You've done it in work situations where you stood up for an unpopular policy and made yourself heard. You've turned away from the married man's advances, even though he was to die for.

I'm trusting you to care for yourself, your appearance, projecting your personal self in the most loving way. I'm going to help you get dressed knowing what's good for you, because getting dressed is a loving act, a creative experience, a party that you can have with yourself every single day.

When you look at a well-dressed woman, you don't think about what she spent on that pair of shoes or how old her dress is. You look at that woman and you see her radiance. She lights up. She stands out.

Every single thing she put on that morning, every color, fabric, and product brought her

radiance

to the fore so we could see it. She is radiant on the inside, and she's dressing to make her radiance compelling on the outside.

That's what I want to teach you, to dress from the inside out. I'm convinced that you know more about yourself now than you did at twenty, that your life experiences have woven a unique tapestry rich in design. Clothes can help express that. We are here on this planet to understand ourselves and others, to learn about love and express it, to *listen to the creativity in our hearts* and to bring it out into our lives.

How amazed you are going to be. By paying attention to getting dressed, you will feel like a renewed version of yourself, updated, revised, and improved. You're already terrific. You're about to get a better view of that, from your closet to your bedroom mirror, from the inside out.

Dress for the Body You Are Currently In

You have to accept whatever comes and the only important thing is that you meet it with courage and with the best that you have to give.

~ELEANOR ROOSEVELT, ESSAY IN *THIS I BELIEVE*, EDWARD P. MORGAN, ED. 1953

EVERYBODY'S GOT A BODY. For four decades, yours has been growing, changing, and regenerating. From the moment you were born, your body has had a loving plan to serve you the best it can. Tirelessly, fearlessly, it's been there for you. Celebrate it, accept it, now, just as it is, today. Take a good look at it in the mirror, slide your hand over every inch of it that you can reach, and thank it profusely for being the trooper that it's been. Vow today to not put off enjoying it and dressing it deliciously as it is now.

From the age of thirty-eight on, we tend to look in the mirror and see our grandmother's arms. This is an illusion. They are your arms. Bless them. Adorn them lovingly. They serve you well. Forgive yourself for the incessant comparing and contrasting you've put your body through.

When you're focused too tightly on someone's narrow definition of perfection, give yourself a break—just go on an observation picnic. Give your eyes a bath. Watch people. Observe sizes, shapes, features. Your shape and size is one of a gazillion combos. Isn't it amazing how we're all so different? Life would be enormously boring and flat if everyone looked like Cindy Crawford, Sophia Loren, or Marilyn Monroe. Diversity makes the world rich, textural. We need all shapes, colors, and sizes.

Dress the body you are in now.

Don't demand that it be the body you were in five years ago, ten years ago, the one you see in a picture in a magazine. Your body is begging to be adorned beautifully right now. Nothing is wrong with it. You aren't waiting for anything. You're expressing yourself fully now. Don't delay the pleasure of looking and feeling great in clothes because you're not the size you've decided you must be before you indulge your senses in garments that love your body exactly as it is. Depriving yourself here only leads to depression.

Get comfy with your body by getting curious. Strive for understanding. Learn what it wears well. Start by deciding where you want to put the focus. Starting at your head and working down the full length of your body, take a kind inventory. What do you want to bring attention to? What do you find challenging? What needs a little math in order to be in better proportion? Put it on paper objectively. Face, neck, shoulders, arms, hands, back, bust, rib cage, waist, tummy, derriere, thighs, legs, feet. You have plenty of opportunity to use fashion to focus on any of those areas. Put the focus on your assets. Wear colors that match your eyes, necklines with strong defined lines like your strong cheekbones and strong jawline. If you have a beautiful neck, wear open collars or nestle a pretty necklace against your skin. Wear a strong nail polish color to draw attention to your hands, close-fitting tops to follow your strong back. Show some cleavage in a scoop neck T-shirt with your jeans, tuck a shirt into your flat front pants and add a belt to show off your waist. Highlight your great legs in slim pants, terrific arms in a sheer long-sleeved blouse over a tank top, cute adorable feet in skimpy strappy sandals. It's easy! Direct the attention where you want attention and your perceived challenges will disappear into the background. When you highlight your pretty lips with a great lipstick color, your thighs will quiet down and assume their proper proportions.

Ignore all numbers on hang tags. You want good fit because good fit is always what flatters. Numbers don't. On one shopping trip, a client bought clothing in sizes 6, 8, 10, and 12—and they were all a perfect fit. Numbers are meaningless. Your body is not a number. It is a form. It only wants to be honored in clothes that fit right.

Size 10
Maybe 8

If you try on something in a dressing room and it doesn't fit your body, it's the fault of the garment, not your body. It's not cut for you. In the olden days, dressmakers traveled from house to house, took measurements, and then produced clothes that fit those specific bodies. Current ready-to-wear takes its best shot at producing clothes that will fit bodies, but if you did your people watching, you realize what a tough assignment that is. One designer's "model" (think dress form) may be for a body that is more narrow, not one that is full, or vice versa. That's why you go up a size with one vendor and down a size with another to get the right fit.

Never declare your body wrong for something not fitting you properly. Keep trying on clothes until you find what makes your body feel happy and joyous. Make friends with a good seamstress or alterations person. These talented professionals understand about bodies and fit and know how to tweak clothes so they perfectly satisfy you. Demand it.

Paint Your Life

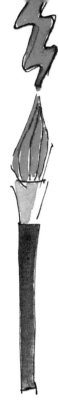

*Know, first, who you are; and
then adorn yourself accordingly.*

~EPICTETUS, *DISCOURSES*

7

AN ARCHITECT DESIGNS A HOME once she's studied the land and what surrounds it. She explores her client's lifestyle. Then she draws up a blueprint that responds to the needs and pleasures of the people who will live there. She wants that home to work completely, so she asks lots of questions ahead of time. She considers all the information before plans are drawn, approved, and ground is broken.

In order to have a wardrobe that responds quickly and completely to all the demands for clothes in your life, you need to ask yourself lots of questions and come up with a current blueprint of your life. This chapter and the next three will help you develop your blueprint. Then, when you start working with the clothes in your closet or in stores, you will be confidently armed with self-defining information to create a mind-blowing success with clothes.

You've been a lot of places, done a lot of things. I honor the journey you took to get here, but let's get current. Look at the calendar. I'm interested in defining who are you today — on this date, this month, in this year. If you were making a pie chart that represented your life today, what would be in there? Are you a mother, lover, friend, aunt, wife, sister, godparent? Are you a caretaker of elderly parents, a student, a scholar, a traveler, an athlete? Are you a businesswoman, an entrepreneur, an employee, an employer? Have you left the corporate life and switched to a home office? Are you entering the work force after a break? Are you an actor, painter, teacher, doctor, nurse, volunteer? What "hats" do you wear? Before we look at clothes, I want you to look at your life on paper. You'll be able to see it more clearly this way. By getting current, you won't waste money or time buying clothes for a past life.

Roles/Activities Exercise: Take a blank piece of paper. On the left-hand side, list all your roles, the "hats" you currently wear. On the right-hand side, list the activities these roles incorporate. If one of your roles is "painter," your paper might look like this:

Role	Activities
painter	painting in studio
	presenting portfolio to perspective clients
	visiting art galleries and museums
	sketching in nature
	meeting with gallery owners

You can see that one role can require several different appropriate sets of clothing. You may spend most of your time in the studio in paint-splattered denim overalls, but you'll pull out the silk suit and heels for your opening reception.

Write out every detail of your life. What are you wearing clothes to and for? You are interviewing yourself, gathering the material to prepare a blueprint so as architect of your wardrobe, you will have thought of everything that needs to go into this award-winning, awe-inspiring wardrobe that always works for you.

Gathering information may flush out some areas of your life that you had forgotten. Our painter may have overlooked the outfit that she needs to wear once a month when meeting bank executives who are considering her paintings for their offices.

Needs/Wants Exercise: Keeping your roles and activities in mind, proceed to this next query. Put these two questions at the top of a blank piece of paper:

What Do I Need from My Clothes?   *What Do I Want My Clothes to Do?*

_____   _____

_____   _____

_____   _____

_____   _____

_____   _____

_____   _____

_____   _____

_____   _____

_____   _____

_____   _____

Think of every possibility. Topple the walls of what you think you can expect and let your mind dream up answers effortlessly. Do you want your clothes to entertain you or others, to make an impression, to communicate an ideal or value? Be bold in your requests. Do you have a public self that needs grooming? A private image that craves sensual satisfaction and expression? Write it all down, everything you need and want from your clothes at this stage of your life. Don't be shy.

Sally, a forty-year-old professional, wife, and mother, made the following response:

- I want to feel good and be comfortable.
- I want to make a statement about who I am.
- I want to be interesting and distinctive.
- I want to show taste and sophistication and to be beautiful.
- I don't want to make a million trips to the cleaners.
- I want to look in the mirror and say, "Yeah, that's me and I look good!"
- I want to show facets of myself and show my depth of personality.
- I don't want to look fussy or contrived.

Here's forty-one-year-old Anna's response:

- As a mother, I need my clothes to work for me and still convey that I am totally together.
- As a CEO wife, I need my clothes to say "confident, sophisticated" but also "accessible, warm, and caring."
- As a volunteer, I need to look like I'm on the cutting edge.
- As a professional in transition, I need to look like I know where I'm going and that I can meet the challenge—I'm already there.
- As a date, I need to look as exciting as I feel, as loved and as loving—soft, chic, romantic, and self-confident.

Clothes are like puppy dogs. They want to please you like crazy, make you deliriously happy, make you feel like the most special person in the world. They want to love you from the moment you open your eyes in the morning to the minute you walk through the door at night. All they ask of you is to figure out what you truly need and want from them. Like teaching points in any communication course you've taken, one of your primary tasks is to figure out what the heck you want so your wishes have a chance to come true. You can't keep it to yourself. Bring it out in the open. Right now; you only have to get it out on paper. Nothing else is required.

Give yourself a quiet moment to do this exercise, quickly, freely. Do it again three days from now and then again as often as you like until it feels complete, like everything that wants to be said and acknowledged has found its way to the page. Then sit back and take it in. This may be the first time you've let yourself know what you really want. You are getting current information about yourself.

Celebrate!

This is all good.

Stop Whining and Go Do Your Homework

It is the soul's duty to be loyal to its own desires.
It must abandon itself to its master passion.

~REBECCA WEST, QUOTED IN
GLIMPSES OF THE GREAT

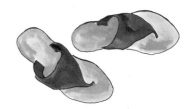

8 GREAT. HOW'S YOUR BLUEPRINT COMING ALONG? I trust that you have not put one boot, mule, tennis shoe, sandal, oxford, or pump into a store yet. You have not spent one dollar on clothes. I don't want to hear any whining from you about "Why can't I go shopping yet?" You're still defining where you are and where you're headed, so shopping is the last place for you right now. Instead, I hope you are getting dressed in your same clothes every morning but with some new awareness. You're thinking about what you wrote down in your Needs/Wants Exercise, and you're taking a look to see if your clothes are living up to what you want from them. If they aren't, that's great. You're seeing the gap between what you want and what you have. You're realizing that your wardrobe doesn't match your current roles and activities, that you've got lots of clothes in your closet from past lives. Good.

I want to spend more time in that gap between what works and what doesn't because that's where all the ripe possibilities live. You can't take a leap until you know what spot you're leaping from and what direction you want to be leaping toward. I want you to clearly see where you are (what your starting point is) and where you want to be (your desired ending point) so you can recognize it clearly when you get there. Are you with me? Okay. You're ready for the next homework assignment.

Moving Away From/Moving Toward Exercise: Get out another piece of paper. On the top left write "Moving Away From." On the top right, put "Moving Toward."

Now think about your clothes, the state of your closet, how you get dressed, your current style or lack of it, what is working and what's not. Comparisons might be illuminating here. Think about your friends or sisters and what you covet about their clothes, style, closets, appearance. What do they do well that you would love to have in your life? You're paying tribute to them. This isn't about jealousy or envy. You're being more objective than that. And you're also not beating yourself up when you're talking about what you're moving away from.

It's okay if these problems have been around as long as soap flakes. You're just stating facts. What is it in the realm of clothes and getting dressed that you'd really like to move away from? And what is it you would like to move toward? Don't censor anything, no matter how far-fetched it seems to you. This exercise helps you find out where you're starting from and where you're headed so you have a greater chance of getting there. The following examples will help you get started:

From forty-eight-year-old Sally:

Moving Away From	*Moving Toward*
being invisible	being powerful
hiding, withdrawing	brilliance, elegance, boldness
not wanting to wear anything in my closet	wearing everything

From forty-two-year-old Debra:

Moving Away From	*Moving Toward*
tradition	being who I am
structured, stiff	creative expression
a closet with clothes I don't wear	happy choices
looking good once in awhile	looking consistently great
looking tired, boring	looking vibrant, playful
accessory terror	knowing how to use accessories

From forty-five-year-old Kerry:

Moving Away From	*Moving Toward*
being too efficient	being more relaxed
plainness	special
not having to buy the same trousers in every single color	being open-minded; more solutions exist than I know

From forty-five-year-old Ellen:

Moving Away From	*Moving Toward*
confusion	having fun with clothes
boring	wow, arty, edgy, rockin'
"it doesn't quite work"	ability to walk in and know "Boom! it works"

It's easy to see by reading other women's personal responses that we're all different. You may relate to some of them but have other issues. Put your issues on paper! They have to see the light of day to shift from what you have and don't want to what you do want.

These aren't new principles. I'm sure you've experienced them in other areas of your life, maybe in major life-altering ways. You realize you want to live a creative, expressive life (Moving Toward). Your current life holds a family and marriage that revolves around everyone else but you, meets everyone else's needs but yours (Moving Away From). There's a gap between the two. With your focus on what you want to move toward, many creative solutions present themselves. Possibilities may include going back to school, setting up an artist's studio with studio hours that you faithfully keep for yourself, or attending college career exploration classes. It may include divorce and starting over in an environment conducive to your personal expression.

You may be surprised at how deeply you will commit to change once you've fully identified what you want to move away from. No more accepting the status quo, no more repeating mistakes, no more covering up your beauty and radiance. It's time for a change! By doing this exercise, you can see what direction will take you toward that change. Once you've declared what the future will look like, life's creative forces and wisdom can leap in to carry you forward.

Love Is All There Is

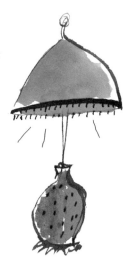

9 THERE'S A BIG OLE LOVE FEST going on inside of you. It wants to come out and be a part of your everyday life, to be expressed in the clothes you wear and everything that you have around you. What do you love? No one knows but you. You may have some loved ones who have some insight, but don't call on them yet. I want you to be the one to pick up the shovel and do the groundbreaking on this project.

I can hear you now. You know just how your daughter Jennifer likes her scalloped potatoes. You know the shade of blue that your friend Patrick thrives on. You know the sock style your husband can't live without — over the calf, black, basketweave knit. You're the expert on your family's preferences. You hold the key to their pleasure zones. But what about yours? I bet your knowledge of what curls your own toes is more limited. How do I know? Am I psychic? No, this is one of those no-brainers. You're a woman, forty or more. You know exactly what floats everyone else's boat. You're a little shaky about what floats yours.

Put everyone else aside for a minute and just think about yourself. I want you to search your precious soul and discover everything you can about what thrills you. Your next assignment is mandatory enrollment in Love Boot Camp, where you'll follow orders and study love—your love. You're going to eat, drink, and breathe love. Don't even think about wiggling out of this step or slipping down to the mall for some recreational shopping. Not yet! You'll get nowhere unless you do this step. It's not calculus, but I want you to concentrate as if it were. The key to your happiness in clothes is to discover what you love today. I want an up-to-the-minute report. It's not the same as when you were twenty-five. And it's not the same as when you were thirty-five. Time has marched on and so has your style and your love patterns. They've evolved, even while you weren't noticing.

If you're squirming, edgy, or impatient, put it aside and recommit to further exploration of the fascinating subject of you. You're probably not used to putting the spotlight on yourself. You are, after all, a woman. Don't worry. Discomfort is not terminal. You will survive Love Boot Camp. Now hop to and let's get going.

Here's where you start. Curl up with a stack of magazines that you have bought, stolen, or borrowed. You're going to be ripping these up. They can be fashion magazines or clothing catalogs, or gardening, decorating, or architecture publications — just about anything that has pictures. Give yourself minutes, hours, days, or weeks to go through these magazines. Look at the ads as well as the editorial/photo layouts, and rip out anything that you adore. It could be a color combo of turquoise, red, and bright yellow. It could be an ensemble of subtle shades of one color — cool greens that range from moss green to a dusty olive green. Maybe it's a room where everything is white and you love its quiet beauty. Rip out the picture. Maybe it's the offbeat way a scarf is worn, or the contrast of two ornate bangle bracelets on an arm contrasted with simple clothing. Maybe it's the rough texture of fabrics, or the shimmer of fabrics. Maybe it's a mood, a picture of a flowery, lacy Victorian room that sends you. Or maybe it's sleek, cool, hard-edged contemporary, chunky jewelry that thrills you. Make notes on the pages or on sticky notes to remind you of what you loved. It may be just a portion of a picture.

What to do: Ignore all price tags. Remember, you aren't buying these things, so if the caption says the ring you're swooning over is $14,000, that's okay.

What not to do: Don't fail to pull out a picture because you say to yourself, "Well, I couldn't wear that anyway." This isn't about wearing, it's about loving. Visually loving.

After you have exhausted magazine ripping, sit down with your pictures and spread them out. You can invite a friend to be a witness and an assistant at this stage. Or invite several of them and do this for each other. Now look at each picture and describe what you love about it. If you're doing this with a friend, have your friend jot down key words on an easel or in a notebook. One at a time, tell what you love about each picture. If you're doing this alone, listen to yourself and take your own notes. Halfway into this, you may start to see a theme. Group the pictures together that demonstrate that theme. It might involve a consistent passion for bright colors or for smooth fabrics and very clean, quiet, elegant design. You could have a run of pictures that are full of whimsy.

Be a detective. Identify the evidence before you. Do you like real girly details—ruffles, lace, bows? Or do you like straight, clean lines? Do you like bright colors or soft, muted colors—sand, eggshell, mushroom, bark? Do you like shiny, crisp fabrics? Or did you pick pictures that mixed all kinds of patterns and fabrics?

If you picked out interior pictures, talk about their quality. If you have three pictures of rooms that are all white, you might love the quiet of monochromatic outfits, dressing head to toe in one color, such as beige or cream. If your interior pictures were country houses with lots of wood and cozy overstuffed chairs and sofas and patterns all around in quilts and throws, your detective might point out the informality of the scenes, the comfort, the unpretentiousness, the ease. In clothing that could mean casual, easy fabrics—denim, cotton knits, plaid shirts or jackets, short boots, soft tote bags, leather or suede jackets. You're not a candidate for prim and proper, neat and tidy gabardine suits, silk blouses, and shiny shoes.

If you selected pictures of gardens, look at their attributes. Is yours a classic garden with very neat rows, well-tended? You might absolutely love classic looks in clothes. A fan of wild, overgrown English gardens may like mixing several elements into an ensemble, wearing different textures or mixing patterns together in a loose way.

Listen closely to the words you've used to describe your pictures. Can you see how those words speak about you? These specific qualities are ingredients in the recipe of your style. If you saw a few main themes and then had a couple of extraneous pictures that were completely different from the others, a couple of things could be going on. Eighty percent of your style may be consistent, but then you've got a "motorcycle mama" that needs to come out once in a while. You might have several pictures of black leather pants and jackets, bright red lipstick, and big clunky boots. It's part of you. It belongs in your group of pictures if you currently resonate with that. If it's from the past and you honestly ask yourself, "Is this current?" the answer may be no. If the answer is no, toss that picture in the trash. We want the up-to-the-minute pulse on what wants to be expressed in you.

You'll need a folder—not any old folder; one that you treasure—or a three-ring binder with plastic sleeve protectors where you'll store these pictures that you've collected. Sometimes when you first pull pictures, you worry that you won't have enough, so you pick things that are okay but not ones that you are weak-kneed in love with. Throw those "just okay" pictures out. Save only the ones that you are truly smitten with, even if it's just five pictures. Sometimes one picture can really nail the qualities that point to your personal style and its expression. Keep a page in your notebook with your notes and the key elements of your style.

Keep building and refining this style portfolio. Add to it each season. Remove pictures that no longer resonate with you. Keep it pure. They're really valuable to remind yourself of who you are, who you've become. They will inspire you to create what you see in them. The reason you did this exercise was to identify what you love so you can have it all around you. Keep referring to these pure expressions.

"My Favorite Things" Exercise: Here's an exercise that will elicit more words or phrases to help you zero in on your personal style.

Pick out three things that you are deliriously crazy about. They could be knick-knacks, art, jewelry, a vase. Anything you especially love. One by one look at each object, and then talk about it. Again, take notes or have a friend do it for you. What is it that makes you so fond of these objects? Listen to how you describe these love objects. Write it all down. Look at your words on the page. Can you make a connection between what you've written and your clothes?

One woman adored her whimsical, colorful tea kettle. She loved its strong, rich colors—burnt orange, red, teal, leaf green, and gold. All of these colors looked glorious on this redhead. In fact, color became a major ingredient of her identifiable style. That tea kettle became her color palette. The same thing happened with Kim. We were able to lift her whole color scheme from a multicolored Persian rug that she loved voraciously. The rug's colors all looked great on her.

Sandy loved a wide bracelet made from a cluster of antique buttons. What did she appreciate about it? "I love the idea of something old—the buttons are from the forties or fifties—put into a modern design. I like the mix of the old and the contemporary." For Sandy, distinctive jewelry became a signature item of hers. She is not a woman who wears fine gold jewelry. It would look ridiculous on her. She likes dressing in modern fabrics, modern clothes (the new) but with a piece of antique jewelry. Her clothes can be modern, but her accessories need to be from another era. This totally satisfies her design sense, her personal style.

Okay, what have you learned about yourself in Love Boot Camp? What three things can you declare about your style recipe? I know you saw some patterns emerge. What were they? Whatever surfaces from your stay at Love Boot Camp will be different from whatever surfaces for your sister or your best friend. **Bask in your uniqueness.**

To Thine Own Self Be True

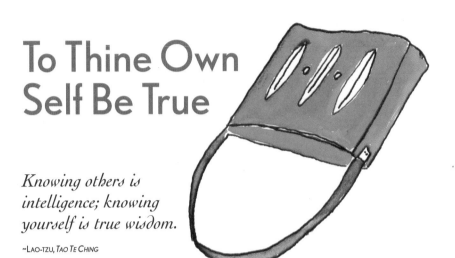

Knowing others is intelligence; knowing yourself is true wisdom.

~LAO-TZU, *TAO TE CHING*

10 THERE'S NO ONE WORTH BEING in the whole wide world but yourself. Be all you, 100 percent you, all the time. In order to do that, we need to interview—*you!* We'll start off easy—with what you like and don't like, in other words, your personal preferences.

It's important to do this next exercise with attitude. Although it's the "What I Like/What I Don't Like" exercise, you can amp it up to "What I Love/What I Hate." Get passionate about this! Be like a teenager and stand for your opinions in a big way. On the top left side of a big sheet of paper write "What I Like (Love)" and on the top right side write "What I Don't Like (Hate)."

When my oldest daughter was eight, she was asked

whether or not she liked a certain food. She answered, "I kinda like it, but I mostly hate it." As a teenager, she's not nearly as demure as that. If you mostly hate something, put it in that column. Sometimes it's easier to recognize what we like by first dumping out what we don't like. And if you kinda like it, skip it. Go to something you're more adamant about. Don't be nice or tactful. Be brutally honest.

What are you giving your hot-headed opinions about in this exercise? I want you to spill out whatever comes to your mind, both general and specific, about clothes, types of clothes, accessories, color, textures, patterns, details, weights of fabrics, everything you can think of. Do you like solid colors, smooth fabrics, body-skimming lines, hardly any accessories, and hate plaid, floral prints, ruffles, epaulets, bulky fabrics, and anything fussy? Do you like a casual look, or do you prefer a more formal style? Do you enjoy clothes or accessories with designer labels, or do you hate that kind of thing? Do you like to feel covered up, or do you love to be more revealing? Do you seek to blend in, or do you like to stand out? You also have preferences when it comes to things like home furnishings, places to vacation, entertainment, book genres, art, music, and food. They all contribute to creating the picture of who you are. Look at how you put your home together. Is it cozy, casual, full of warm woods, fresh flowers, and patterned throw pillows everywhere? Or is it more formal, with antique, dark, high-gloss furniture, cut-crystal vases, pictures framed in shiny metal frames, quiet landscapes on the walls? Your preferences in your home reflect your personal style, which in turn can be translated into your clothes style.

Remember this infamous Barbara Walters interview question that came at the end of her interviews with top celebrities? "If you were a tree, what kind of tree would you be and why?" As simplistic as that sounds, I want you to answer a similar question in this interview with yourself. If you were a type of flower, what flower would you be, and what is it that you love about that type of flower? Would you be like a daisy because it's fresh, unassuming, clean, simple? Would you be a rose—beautiful to look at but hard to get close to? Would you be a bromeliad because it's hearty, beautiful, and exotic? Stop snickering and dive into this exercise. Write as much as you can about that flower and see whether there aren't some words or phrases that come out of it that help give words to your style sense. That daisy lover may have a personal style that is "fresh, unassuming, clean, and simple." Those words can gracefully guide her in designing her personal style. See if it works that way for you.

Because it's often much easier to identify things about other people than it is to do so for ourselves, do the "Pick a Fashion Hero" exercise next. Think about someone whose style you really admire—a friend, an acquaintance, a celebrity that you only know through pages of magazines. Don't get hung up on the fact that she may be very different from you in size, age, looks, and other attributes. Just study what you like about her style. By identifying what she does well, you are hitting upon a fashion philosophy that might translate into some things you like for yourself.

One of my fashion heroes is a petite forty-six-year-old woman who has, as far as I can tell, ignored all the "petites" rules to dress taller. Instead she dresses for her personal style. She has special interests in art that are congruent with how she dresses. She's approachable, yet sophisticated, very modern. She playfully wears a loosely woven white textured sweater and contrasts it with a black textured scarf, which is like adding MSG to food—the contrast of colors enhances the texture. She's always pulled together, yet you can expect at least one thing to be unexpected about her—the way she's pulled her hair back, her variety of reading glasses that add spice to her outfits, a kicky pair of shoes with a more tailored suit. As I write about her, I can easily extract a few key phrases that resonate with me, things I'd like to express in my personal style— arty, sophisticated, whimsical, attention to detail, every piece of the ensemble working together. I can take these qualities that I admire in her and see how I might apply them to myself.

During the Renaissance, aspiring artists worked as apprentices and studied the masters by directly and meticulously copying masterworks. They learned how wonderful paintings were put together, and then they went on to make their own mark—like Michelangelo did. Studying and identifying what you really admire will give you information that you can then apply to develop and enhance your own personal style.

The more you honor your preferences and wear those preferences or looks, the more saturated your self-expression will be. That's what I'm aiming for—a 100-proof expression of you. Here's how to tell if you're close to doing that. **Take this test every morning:** Look in the mirror. If you are wearing clothes that reflect you, your life, and your personality, then your diaphragm will relax, you will sigh and take **pleasure in what you see.**

If you are dressed in clothes (or a look) that's not right for you, you will look and feel like you're in someone else's clothes, like you are wearing a costume.

Look Like Yourself

*I'm talking about a little truth in packaging here. To be
perfectly frank, you don't quite look like yourself. And if
you walk around looking like someone other than who
you are, you could end up getting the wrong job,
the wrong friends, who knows what all. You could end
up with somebody else's whole life.*

~MICHAEL CUNNINGHAM,
A HOME AT THE END OF THE WORLD

11 I STOPPED FOR A RED LIGHT at the
corner of Post and Powell in San
Francisco. I glanced at the tall
woman standing next to me at
the crosswalk. She carried an
unusual greeny-gray shiny
leather handbag tucked under
her arm. She was otherwise
dressed head-to-toe in black wearing a
classic jacket and slim, short skirt. I was mesmerized. She was
our age. She looked so great, what was it about her? As I studied her for the couple of minutes before the light turned green,
I realized her handbag was the same difficult-to-describe color

as her eyes, I mean, *exactly* the same color. And her hair was the darkest brown-black, which was duplicated in the color of her suit. She wore nude hose with tall black pumps. It was so right. She could have carried a turquoise handbag and worn a coral suit and I probably never would have spent a minute looking at her. She caught my eye because she was copying in her clothes part of the pattern that her own natural coloring created.

When you copy yourself, you come into focus, you leave a lasting impression, you put yourself in the best light. When you look at someone and you know they're doing something really right, there's a reason. When you study them, you'll see the relationship between who they are and what they're wearing.

Let me give you some more examples of this. I knew a woman who wore thin hoop earrings nearly every day, and they looked perfect on her. When I studied her face, I saw that her eyebrow line was that same thin width as her earring.

I was taken by the looks of a woman with curly strawberry-blond hair. She seemed to have a trademark of wearing patterned scarves in her hair that were always a little off-kilter — just like every one of her features. She had a crooked smile, a crooked eye, lots of asymmetry in her face. Finding a way to create asymmetry in her accessories was a way to create "balance" in her. The patterned scarves repeated the pattern of her curly hair. It was brilliant.

Paloma Picasso several years back had an ad campaign for her jewelry line that ran in all the fashion magazines. Her jewelry was bold, large-scale, very dramatic — exactly like Paloma Picasso's looks. She had jet-black, straight hair, strong large-scale features. The jewelry was congruent with her looks. Had she been seen in a little seed-pearl necklace and dangly earrings, she would have looked ridiculous.

You probably copy yourself instinctively, but see if you can do it on purpose: Take a close look at yourself and see how you can relate your physicalness to your clothes. Here are some ways to look like yourself. If you have thick hair, wear fabrics that look like they have a "thickness" to them. Really thin fabrics will look funny on you unless you layer them. For instance, you can wear a thin, silk chiffon scarf if it has a lot of width and it bunches up and appears "thick" when you put it around your neck. A woman with thin, short hair could be overwhelmed by this and would naturally prefer something narrower.

Someone with a real ruddy complexion—freckled or weathered or wrinkled—would enjoy fabrics that mirror her patterning. She might like a tweed or nubby fabric with surface texture rather than a perfectly smooth, flat shiny fabric like a silk charmeuse.

Repeat your coloring like the woman at the crosswalk. Are your eyes azure blue or smokey blue, jade, golden brown? Repeat your unique eye color in sweaters, T-shirts, blouses, jackets. You may build a wardrobe around your eye color. If you have a lot of contrast in your coloring, your hair brown/almost black, your skin fair, your eyes dark brown, repeat your color pattern in clothes with highly contrasting colors—black and white together. If you haven't had your colors charted, discovering what really enhances your natural coloring could be an eye-opener. The right colors make you look healthy and beautiful.

With the changes in coloring that happen after forty, it's essential that you keep up with your shifting tableau. The gray in your hair, the extra line or two on your face creates new patterns and textures just waiting to be enjoyed. You may fall in love with shades of gray, discovering the beauty of mixing in various textures to create interest. Wear charcoal slacks with a pearl-gray silk charmeuse blouse with a natural luster that gets you out of drab-dom. Add a medium-gray cashmere shawl and you're showing off one of your new best colors. Add more pattern and texture in your clothes to welcome home the new design that forty brought.

When you're dressing from the inside out, it's important to bring out some inside qualities that could be missed. Ask yourself: What do people know about me right off the bat? What's not obvious but that you'd like people to know about you without having to tell them? If you are someone that everyone comes to with their troubles and you'd rather be known for your irreverence, wear accessories that are playful: a bracelet that looks like a cluster of grapes or a silk scarf with fruit as a motif. Wear wild socks, a mix of bright colors, have two-weeks' worth of polka-dotted shirts in your closet. Wear irreverent.

If you're someone who's "cute as a button," you may have to set the record straight and let people know that you're also very smart and you want to be respected for those smarts. Take all the froufrou out of your wardrobe. Dress in messages of authority—darker colors, smooth fabrics, no pattern. Clothing has messages built into it, so be sure you're saying what you want to be saying about yourself. Let me tell you about some of clothing's messages.

Clothing Messages

Color Speaks: Navy, gray, black, and other dark shades say professional, authoritative, "I mean business." Light, bright colors, especially when two or more are put together give a message of playfulness, casualness, "We're having fun now!"

Texture's Story: Smooth fabrics in tight weaves say, "I'm efficient, professional; I'll get the job done." Nubby tweeds, loose weaves, mixing and matching textures is more friendly, approachable, cozy.

Pattern Tells All: Little or no pattern is more serious, authoritative; big abstract prints (think Hawaiian shirts) say fun, fun, fun; little floral prints say, "I'm sweet."

Line Messages: Vertical, straight up and down lines are more formal, rigid. Think pinstripe suits worn in the banking world. Curved, circular, or meandering lines are more playful, sensual, inviting.

Accessories Talk: Shiny gold is most formal, next comes silver. Matte finishes or colored metals are more informal; jewelry made from wood, paper, or fabric is taken less seriously and is not seen as very important.

How you combine color, texture, pattern, line, and accessories directly affects how you're perceived. Playing with these elements is like creating new recipes. If you're in a situation where you need others to see your professional self, line up all those ingredients. When you're bringing out your playful self to socialize, send yourself and your audience that message in what you choose to wear. If you're in a creative work setting, go ahead and team that Hawaiian-type shirt with your navy-blue linen suit for the right mix of serious and informal messages. Be yourself—on purpose.

Clothes Are Like Food

It has long been an axiom of mine that the little things are infinitely the most important.

~SHERLOCK HOLMES, QUOTED IN
A GENTLEMAN'S WARDROBE:
CLASSIC CLOTHES AND THE MODERN MAN
BY PAUL KEERS

12 ARE YOU A FAST-FOOD JUNKIE, living on lunch in your car, dinner while standing at the kitchen sink, not really paying much attention to what makes it down your digestive track?

There's also such a thing as the careless clothes junkie, the person who, like the fast-food junkie, is pretty mindless when it comes to dressing. These are often folks who get dumped on. Their sister, friend, or cousin dumps their rejects on them when cleaning out closets. Since the givers like to pass on their mistakes to ease their own guilt, the receiver looks like an orphan (or cold leftovers) in everyone else's rejects. It's not an appetizing sight. Do you have a wardrobe that's just getting by? Not putting a lot of thought or tender care into your clothes?

When you eat at a fine restaurant, a lot of care has gone into the quality of ingredients and the presentation of the meal on the plate that's set before you. It really shows. It's memorable, and you savor that meal for days or months. You can call it up in your memory like a thrilling movie, a favorite beach, or a particular night of great sex.

Great dressing is like that too. Maybe it's the outfit you wore when you first met your husband. Maybe it's the summer dress you were wearing under your gown the day you graduated from college. What outfits can you recall from your past? I remember a pantsuit in a languid fabric, a periwinkle-blue tunic and floaty pants, a long print scarf in silk satin with fringe at the ends that looked great any which way it hung around my neck or shoulders, and the sweet mules that I slipped into. It was a special party. Christie remembers the ensemble she wore to her son's wedding. She was head-to-toe in soft gold tones, from her wide brimmed hat to her simple silk sheath dress, her shimmering gold jacket, and her simple golden pumps. She was a picture in different finishes of the same color, from matte gold in her dress to the shiniest gold of her jacket.

What do you remember? Was it the presentation—how the main outfit was accessorized or garnished—that made it look so great? Was it the quality of the dress, something you splurged on, like you would a dinner at a fine restaurant?

To create memorable scintillating outfits, focus on quality ingredients.

Quality ingredients in a salad make it a thrill to eat. Wilted lettuce or brown radishes kill an appetite. Adding unusual ingredients to a salad—star fruits (carambola), golden beets sliced thin and scalloped along the edges, golden peppers instead of green ones—makes it exotic and exciting. What ingredients can you add to your ensemble that will make it delicious to look at? Adding an antique amber necklace, where all the heart-shaped pieces glisten invitingly, can make your ensemble especially exciting. Have various appetizing accessories ready to garnish your outfits. It could be jewelry bought on your travels, estate jewels, scarves collected from artists who sell their works in art galleries. Look for unique accessories to make your outfits original and memorable.

Quality fabrics are delectable. Not only are they beautiful to look at, but they are glorious to wear. The soft hand of a cashmere sweater or the lovely weight of a tropical wool in a simple dress, the velvet scarf backed in silk charmeuse, the butter leather jacket—yummy! Dress yourself in clothes that feel good to the touch.

Creativity marks a good presentation. The pop of color from a buttercup leather shoulder bag crossing over a warm taupey-gray suit reminds me of the just-right cluster of flowers donning a well-dressed table. Fingernail polish color that picks up a spring leather jacket's iridescent palomino color is delightful. Crisp, well-defined details makes an outfit stand out and be remembered.

When you've assembled your outfit and added the finishing touches, savor your reflection in a full-length mirror. Don't rush out the door. You may wear as many outfits in a day as you eat meals in a day. Every day is different, so soak in the beauty of this day's creations. It's good for your heart.

Have you been to restaurants where they serve a little bit of everything from several cuisines? There will be a Mexican dish, some Japanese appetizers, something Cajun, along with the mashed potatoes and gravy. I'm always suspicious of this kind of mixing. I'm more confident going somewhere that specializes in one type of cuisine.

Think of clothes and accessories that way too. Maybe your flavor in clothing is sexy, creative, traditional, eclectic, romantic, sporty, natural. Don't try to be all things at once. Pick a "flavor" and carry it through in an outfit.

Take an Inventory

Where's the man could ease a heart like a satin gown?

~DOROTHY PARKER,
"THE SATIN DRESS"

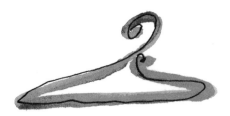

13

TAKING AN INVENTORY is a lot like meal planning and grocery shopping. The more you know about what you need and want, the better chance you have of coming home with it. I hate to admit to the number of times that my family brought in five bags of groceries from the car, put things away, and then looked at each other blankly, realizing we didn't have anything to make for dinner. Besides that, because we didn't take an inventory first, we didn't know about the four family-sized bottles of ketchup, three unopened jars of sage, and two bottles of virgin olive oil already living in the pantry, which meant we didn't need the ones we just bought. I always feel a little foolish and dejected when I've just inefficiently spent a bunch of money.

The same holds true for clothes—only these failures are more expensive than groceries, which makes the remorse deeper and longer lasting. So we're going to prevent that from happening. Taking a clothing inventory will clue you in to the gaps in your wardrobe, so you can make a plan to fill those gaps. That's wardrobe planning.

Give yourself half a day to really poke through your closet like a private detective. I'll suggest several ways to gather clues about your wardrobe. Try them all. The unearthed information will skyrocket you to more success with clothes than you ever dreamed possible.

If you have a portable clothes rack, set it up and start pulling your clothes out of the closet, onto the rack, and into the light of day. With your clothes hanging exposed in your bedroom, you will get a fresh perspective. It's like pulling everything out of the refrigerator to clean it. It's more thorough, and it's easier to see what you've got. Short of a clothes rack, use your bed to lay your clothes out.

Now here's an easy step. Take a head count of the number of suits, skirts, blouses, slacks, and jackets you have. Write down each type of clothing item and the number of them you have. It is illuminating to find out where your multiple bottles of ketchup are. Many people are expert at buying blouses and live years before actually discovering that their wardrobe is made of dozens of blouses and two pairs of slacks, or the opposite. Someone else buys pants all the time but hardly any tops — few sweaters, blouses, T-shirts, or jackets. People often feel more comfortable shopping for half the body; from the waist up or the waist down. Some people have great summer wardrobes but can't figure out how to get through a winter. Become aware of where your muscles are weak, so you can plan for a balanced wardrobe. You may have to put aside your passion for sweaters and do some research on pants, or you'll be complaining about having nothing to wear.

Next start making outfits, complete outfits, from hat to shoes and socks. Try them on and look at yourself in a full-length mirror. Write down these outfits in a wardrobe notebook or on notecards. When you come across the thing you don't have that would complete them, write the name of the item and the outfit it completes on a shopping list. For example,

garnet necklace for plum suit
black close-fitting boots for slim black
    pants and red sweater
olive straight skirt for long tapestry jacket
nude hose for brown plaid suit
two-inch-wide brown belt for jeans

By finishing the outfits you already have a start on, your wardrobe will at least triple once you purchase the items that complete the ensembles. Think of it as a recipe. You have the sugar, flour, and butter, but you're missing the vanilla and chocolate chips. There can't be any warm, yummy chocolate chip cookies without those last items.

As you're sleuthing through your wardrobe, pay close attention to the items that you really abuse—the ivory silk T-shirts, your black oxfords, your camisoles. Recognize these items that are really the glue to your wardrobe. Know that if they disintegrated tomorrow, you truly could not walk out of the house clothed. Add those items to your shopping list, so you have backups before the originals meet their demise.

You may be thinking this sounds too simplistic. Let me share a story with you. Many years ago I was taking a few days to myself at a bed-and-breakfast inn just forty-five minutes from where I live. Over breakfast one of the guests, a university professor from Germany, wanted to know about my business. She was fascinated and told me about her own personal experiment. She loved clothes but never felt put together. So one day she took it upon herself to complete this assignment: Put one outfit together from head to toe. It was very difficult for her to stay with it, but she didn't stop until she had all the ingredients down to the right coat and handbag. She reflected on the process for herself. It involved valuing herself enough to do the project, to be okay with actually having what she yearned for—to be put together and feel good about how she looked, to show up in the world as someone who was "together." I share this with you because you may also experience some epiphanies you didn't expect. You understand the vast difference in eating take-out food from a container in front of the TV versus having a complete meal planned and prepared with grace and served at a dining room table with nice china and silverware. In both cases, it's food, but the latter is nourishing on multiple levels. Having a pulled-together look with no pieces missing is just as nourishing to the body, mind, and spirit as that well-planned meal.

When you're food shopping with a list, the whole event is swift and efficient. When you take an inventory and bring that shopping list with you to the store to finish those clothing recipes that are hanging at home half-baked, two things happen. You can go through a store filled with merchandise, but since you know what you're looking for, you can block out all the useless items and the things you need will practically leap off the racks at you. It's easy!

By shopping for specific
items first, you are hours away
from having a wardrobe that
works right now.
If you get sidetracked and bring
home items not on your list, you're
probably adding more problems,
more unfinished outfits.
Create solutions.
Buy what's on your list first.

What to Buy

Take care to get what you like or you will be forced to like what you get.

~BERNARD SHAW,
MAXIMS FOR REVOLUTIONISTS

THIS IS SIMPLE. Only buy—whether it's underwear, shoes, or a party dress—what you love. Not kinda, not sorta, not "it'll do." Buy what makes your heart sing, what moves you. I want you to lay down in your bed after a shopping trip and be so deliriously pleased about your purchases that you can't sleep. And if you do fall asleep, you'll wake up in the morning and won't be able to wait to slip into your underwear, select your socks, and choose your sweater and pants because everything you have purchased are your favorites. Don't compromise. Don't settle. Be delighted by your key chain, nuts about the color of your wallet, crazy over your kelly-green handbag, wild about your apricot cashmere sweater, cuckoo over your slingback woven sandals.

Fess up. You have a pit in your stomach right now because most of the things hanging in your closet are there because they were close enough, kinda worked, were on sale, you thought they would do in a pinch.

Not anymore. You are going to develop your radar for **YES!**, for looking at something, savoring it with your senses, and knowing that the item in front of you is *the one*.

Sound exhausting? Too much trouble? You are never too much trouble. These items are going to be living with you once you plunk money down on the counter. They are your possessions. You're responsible for them from here on out. Once they've made it through the front door, like kids, it takes a long time, an emotional separation, to get them out. They'll need your care. They'll be staring at you every day when you open your closet door.

Why not have your clothes be the most delightful items you can choose, so everywhere you look, with every decision about getting dressed, you're only experiencing pleasure? Once you develop your radar for **YES!**, it'll be a snap. Feeling shaky about your radar? Let's tackle that first. Somewhere inside of you is a place that knows **YES!** Hands down, without a doubt, **YES!**! Here's a story about **YES!** that my former mother-in-law, Jeanne, told me. She was at a USO dance during World War II with her girlfriend Rosalind. A very handsome man in a uniform came through the front door. Jeanne grabbed her friend's elbow and whispered, "See that man over there? I'm going to marry him." There was no hesitation. She knew, **YES!** Before the night was over, the handsome man, Charley, crossed the dance floor and asked Jeanne to dance. They were married a year later.

What's your **YES!**? Maybe it's not the man you just had to take home with you. Maybe it's something simple like a potted crimson amaryllis in bloom at Christmas that stared you down from a gift store window. Is it a bar of French soap whose smell and color you love? It's round, fits perfectly in your hand. You buy it, bring it home, use it the first time, and swear you're in heaven. That's a **YES!** You don't get the same shiver with Zest, Dove, or glycerin soap.

You saw a scarf that was way too much money, but you bought it anyway because the design was in a leaf pattern and leaves are your thing—you have stationery with leaves, a leaf candy dish, leaves on your bath towels. Every time you wear that scarf, you feel comforted by the design, cuddled by the velvet on one side and the silk on the other side. That scarf is a big **YES!**

What have been some of your **YES!**es? Some of mine are a one-of-a-kind brooch in two parts, the top part a glistening hunk of adamite in a rough heart shape with a piece of faceted topaz hanging from it; a peach lace demi-cup bra from France, a copper bowl with odd little charms hanging off the lip of it; a pair of easy cotton pants with a background pattern of graffiti in the colors of sliced banana bread. After years of service, the brooch, the graffiti pants, and the peach bra have all passed on. They became worn out or broken. The bowl still sits in my office. These things gave me an immense amount of pleasure.

Name three **YES!**es. Keep them vivid in your memory. Now use your **YES!** experience and take that YES! with you when you shop.

Give everything the **YES!** test. You're shopping for

underwear. Buy only **YES!** You need a new pair of rainboots. Take the time to listen for **YES!** You're shopping for jeans. Buy the ones that shout **YES!** When you have on something that is **YES!**, you feel like a queen. You look at yourself and you are joyfully satiated.

The next time you're buying a scarf, really check it out. Touch it, turn it upside down. Slip it around your neck. Does it take your breath away, do you feel your knees go weak, do your cheeks flush, just a little? Does time stop while you're in a reverie of pleasure? If the answer is

YES!,

buy it.

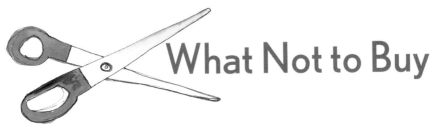

What Not to Buy

*Look here, I have bought this bonnet. I do not think it is
very pretty; but I thought I might as well buy it as not.
I shall pull it to pieces as soon as I get home, and see if
I can make it up any better . . . Oh! but there were two
or three much uglier in the shop; and when I have
bought some prettier-coloured satin to trim it with
fresh, I think it will be very tolerable.*

~THE CHARACTER OF LYDIA BENNET IN
JANE AUSTEN'S *PRIDE AND PREJUDICE*

WHO OF US OUT THERE hasn't done this? Seen an outfit on a
store rack that was a fixer-upper, one that just needed a little
work, and like Lydia Bennet in *Pride and Prejudice*, brought it
home and turned it into a project. Besides the original cost of
the garment, we add more time, more energy, more expense
with—let's get real—slim odds of improving it to that Martha
Stewart level of excellence we saw in our imagination. If you're
a seamstress by trade, your odds are higher, of course. But fix-
it-uppers need to beware. Women with a lot of determination
and creativity probably need to channel that into designing a
garden, building furniture, or planning a vacation, not taking
on needy clothes. Needy clothes need to stay where they are
and not go home with you. Let's look at a few common traps.

Common Traps

The great dress that needs your waist and hips to be a little smaller in order to fit. Project: Lose five pounds.

Don't buy clothes on speculation that you're going to change sizes. You can look great right now in your own size. Leave the dress with required weight loss in the store. Don't bring it home.

The sweater that you kind of like, and if you decide against it, you could give it to your sister. Project: Clothing your siblings.

Your sister really could do this better on her own. You need to be clear about what works for you. Start there before you start clothing people who haven't asked for your assistance.

A great linen suit in a color that looks awful on you. Project: Have it professionally dyed. Or buy a whole new set of makeup to change your coloring so it'll go with the outfit.

When it comes to color and it's wrong-all-wrong, forget it. Don't torment yourself, just walk away. Some professional dry cleaners provide a dye service and will try to get the color you want, but they're smart. They'll ask you to sign a piece of paper that says you pay for this little experiment, Miss Know-It-All, in case it doesn't turn out. I have paid when it didn't turn out. It hurts. In one case, I got the rich brown I wanted in a silk suit that started out as a rosy taupe, but because the thread had polyester in it and wasn't a natural fiber (natural fibers take dye colors), all the stitching turned white. It was impossible to ignore. I never wore it.

And as for the makeup. Do you really want to go through all that trouble? And expense? If a color is making you look sickly, it's going to take a lot of makeup to cover that up. It's a pain in the butt. Don't do it.

A glitzy knit tank top and long metallic pleated knit skirt. Project: Create a lifestyle to go with the outfit.

If you're the natural girl who hikes in the woods, goes to restaurants in jeans, and works at her computer terminal in her nightgown, this outfit could take years to fit into your life. If you can't see yourself wearing it in your current life or in your just-around-the-corner life, leave it alone—even if it's cute and it fits and it's on sale.

A little sheath dress that would fit better if the armholes were higher, the shoulder seam was pulled up so the natural waist was closer to your own waist, the sleeves were shorter, the shoulder pads were removed, the set-in sleeve was moved in about an inch, and darts were put in along the back panel so it would be slimmer looking. Then it would be perfect! Project: A complete overhaul involving extensive alterations charges.

If the in-store tailor can appropriately alter an outfit, okay. But if you're thinking two steps beyond that, you've got a major project on your hands. That yellow light is turning red right now. Stop!

Here's how buying clothing works best. Get your ducks all lined up in a row — **that's color, fit, style, and lifestyle appropriateness.** Money well-spent and clothes well-worn come from buying what fits properly (now), supports your coloring (as is), shows your body off at its best, **and has a purpose in your current life.**

Next time you're tempted to take on an outfit that needs "a little work," go for coffee in a nearby county and think it over.

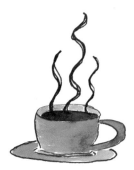

When to Walk Away

You must do the thing you think you cannot do.

~ELEANOR ROOSEVELT, "YOU LEARN BY LIVING"

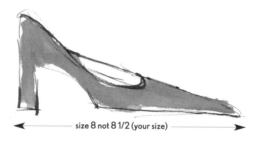

size 8 not 8 1/2 (your size)

16

KNOWING WHEN TO SAY *no* is as powerful as knowing when to say yes. If your *Yes!* radar is a little shaky, then give yourself plenty of space to reach a final decision about purchases. Major department stores and chains offer a more generous return policy than nearly all smaller boutiques. Many stores have a thirty-day return policy. This is plenty of time to see whether an item is going to work for you. You can test your love for it. Does it sustain its intensity after it's home, or does it fade into a ho-hum, non-pulse-raising experience? Remember you're going for *Yes!*

When you're on a mission for a specific item and you're not finding it in the store, walk away. Don't force solutions where there aren't any. New merchandise arrives every week. Ask helpful sales associates about the schedule of arrivals. Try again later.

If you find what you're looking for, but it's not in a flattering color, walk away. Fifty percent isn't enough. Leave the store empty-handed.

Catalog shopping has its appeal, but it's also loaded with downsides. Merchandise is enhanced on glossy pages where well-groomed models are leaning against large boulders on a white sandy beach in Hawaii. When you receive the goods, they're often disappointing. The color isn't true to the photo, the fabric is not the quality that the text and pictures implied. It's inferior more often than it's superior to the sales pages. Then you have to deal with returns. What started out as a convenience becomes very inconvenient when you're filling out return forms, boxing things up, and standing in line at the post office to mail them back. While you're developing your expertise in thoroughly satisfying shopping experiences, there's nothing like having the real thing in your hands or on your body to work with.

If you're familiar with a product and you want it in another color—like a Coach handbag—then go ahead and order it from a catalog. Catalogs are invaluable as sources for ideas. But at the beginning, I want you to get out there and try things on and feel fabrics. I don't want you to lower your standards and settle for merchandise that isn't absolutely right for you. It's too easy to be lazy with catalogs, receive merchandise that isn't right, and then keep it.

Another place to be cautious is the in-home shopping experience where a line of clothing is brought into someone's home or office for a week and women make appointments to check out the merchandise, order what they want in their sizes, color, and fabric, and receive the clothes a few weeks later. This can be a high-pressure setting. You may feel compelled to buy something, even if it doesn't really have a place in your wardrobe plan. And if design is not your passion or vision, choosing fabrics and colors can be really stressful and difficult and too much to take on right now.

Begin right away to build a discerning muscle that helps you shop to please yourself, not a sales clerk on commission, not a friend hosting a home show. Your mission is to have a satisfying, gratifying, effective wardrobe. You are shopping to achieve that, not to please others.

If you have a sales associate who helps you a lot, she's the one that can bend store rules, let you roam around and pull things from other departments into your central dressing room. Use her. She'll bring you water if you're fading. She can hold things for you for a few days if you're feeling overwhelmed and can't make a decision that day.

Remember when you're trying on clothes that 90 percent of what you bring into your dressing room may bomb. Don't get discouraged. Twelve dresses in a row can be awful. That can be useful because when the thirteenth one slips over your head and is gorgeous, it's easier to see by comparison how truly right it is. Don't let numbers of things scare you. Sometimes you try a lot of restaurants before you find the one you love. You date a lot of men before you find Mr. Right. It's the same with clothes. Hold out for the best dress. That's the one you want to walk away with!

Be a quitter when:

- the salesperson just isn't getting it—go to another department or another store rather than listen to someone shoot off their mouth saying all the things you know not to be true—like "that color is great on you" and making you want to throw up
- you're bumming, you're criticizing your body and blaming it instead of recognizing that the garment just isn't right for you
- it's crowded. Shop early in the morning or in evenings from 6 to 9 P.M. for a more relaxed experience
- you're tired, angry, hungry, or lonely. Your decision-making abilities are in the high-risk zone. If you're going to shop under these conditions, then shop only where you can take things back and get a full refund. That way, when you've regained your sense of well-being, you won't be stuck with useless clothing.

Some people swear by retail therapy, shopping to counter depression or other upsets. I'm the kind that can't get out of bed if life is out of step with my plan, so retail therapy has never been an option for me. I have found lots of items in clients' closets that were never worn, still have price tags on them, and were bought during a need for a fix. Shopping may have brought on some temporary relief, but then there's the hangover to deal with when you're looking at what you've purchased and realize these things shouldn't be living with you.

There are other ways to take care of yourself when life sucks: a massage, a matinee, a phone call with a friend. The thing about clothes is once they're home, you have to take care of them too.

If you are shopping to fill a hole that never gets satisfied, or if you have a house where every nook and cranny is stuffed with clothing and it still isn't enough, you need professional help. It's not about clothes anymore. There is a Twelve-Step program called Debtors Anonymous that addresses compulsive shopping. Call information for the phone number of a group near you.

Walk away rather than purchase a pair of to-die-for shoes in a half-size smaller than your normal shoe size, even if they were originally a million dollars and now the store is practically giving them away, unless you plan to use these shoes as coffee table bric-a-brac. You will never wear them. Catch yourself the moment you realize they aren't comfortable, acknowledge your lust, and walk away. You will be a better person for it.

Sales Will Getcha

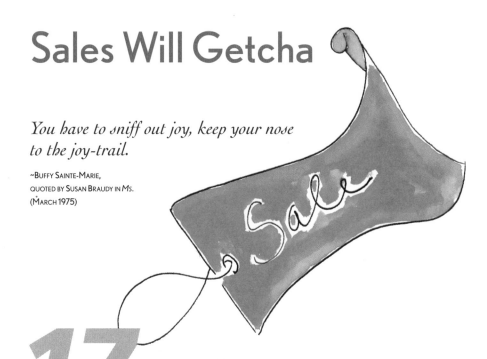

You have to sniff out joy, keep your nose to the joy-trail.

~BUFFY SAINTE-MARIE,
QUOTED BY SUSAN BRAUDY IN *Ms.*
(MARCH 1975)

17

IF SHOPPING ON SALE is your recreational passion *and* you wear and love everything you buy on sale, skip immediately to the next chapter. What I have to say, you've already conquered. If you have bought something on sale and didn't enjoy it much or never wore it, then hunker down and read this chapter twice. It'll save you a carload of money.

Smart women get real dumb in front of a rack of clothes marked 50 percent off. The problem is their IQ drops 50 percent too. Under that sign's shadow, they do things they'd never do if items were full price. They buy a cowboy jacket with fringe that never quite fits into their urban look. They buy spandex pants that a fourteen-year-old should apologize for being seen in. They buy something in the wrong size because, well, it's all that was left, and anyway, it was on sale.

Sales are like drinking. Fess up. You went around the bases much faster with a guy you didn't know that well because of the margaritas, and you never would have even gotten undressed had you been sober.

Shopping during a sale is too often like being inebriated. Your reasoning abilities are grossly affected, your inhibitions lowered. You make excuses for things on sale that you'd never make for items being sold at full price. Your good deal can actually be a very bad deal.

Think about your responses when you're buying something full price. You think it through, you compare and contrast, you see how it works into your plan. You make sober decisions. Your decision is based on the greater vision of your whole wardrobe. You make no excuses.

When you buy on sale, you drop your expectations. It's not quite the right color, *"but it's on sale."* It's not fitting you right, *"but it's on sale."* Although it's a style that looks nice enough, you're not wild about it,

"but it's on sale."

Let's look at value. What is the value to you of looking at a line of clothing at the beginning of a season (at full price) when all the coordinating pieces are available in all the sizes? When everything's there, you may spend half an hour pulling together a capsule wardrobe that works tirelessly for you. What value do you put on your time?

If you shop at the end of the season when things are on sale, what you find in the racks are broken sizes, maybe a size 2, a 4, and a 14 in a jacket. They have two styles of pants, a couple sizes in each style. The skirts flew out the door and there's only one left, a size 16. Putting pieces together to create a working wardrobe is really impossible, although you can spend an afternoon trying.

Consider other things that make it to a sales rack. The department buyer's best guess at what women would be buying for this past season, a best guess that flopped. See all the chartreuse blouses that she thought would get snapped up, but they didn't.

Also on the sale rack are buyer's mistakes from even earlier seasons. Ever notice sometimes how things on the sale rack are things you've never seen before? They could have been the rejects from the Chicago store (and you live in San Francisco). They are a motley-looking bunch of costumes that could be older than your niece. Stores have every right to be trying to unload them. But on you? Damaged goods are on sale too. A rip here, a tear there, a stain on the shoulder.

Are there gems in there, real steals? Probably. For someone. Remember, if you find something that's enticing, but then it needs a skirt and pants to go with it, not to mention shoes and a handbag, that "deal" just cost you a few hundred more dollars to make it work.

Start here first:
You're worth full price.

Read that line again. You're worth full price. Carry that with you and have it handy when you encounter a sale. Use it as a mantra. "I'm worth full price." It'll keep you sober. If you look at the sale item and you're telling yourself you're worth full price, chances are you'll consider whether or not this item has real value for you.

Remember that if you buy a garment in the wrong size, because that's all that was left, you need to figure in your alterations charges before you start celebrating your good fortune.

"Sales" themselves are so common these days that they're frustrating. Are you buying full price and the sale starts tomorrow? Should you shop now or hold out? Should you shop the pre-season sale for your next season clothes or wait until you see what comes in closer to the actual season?

When I was growing up, there used to be two sales—the winter sale that started the day after Christmas and the Crazy Days sale when all the summer sale items would come out on the sidewalk for a weekend in July. It was easy and it was fun to look forward to. No second guessing, no wondering if another chance would come around. Now there are constant sales—the Anniversary Sale, the President's Day Sale, the Super Saturday Sale, the White Flower Day Sale, the Pre-Season Sale, the I-Ran-Over-the-Dog Sale. I mean, really, it's ridiculous. It could be a full-time job staying abreast of the sales, the coupons, and the discount books.

The best thing to do is keep your wits about you. **Shop as if you're paying full price whether you are or not.**

If you bought something and wore the heck out of it, there was tremendous value at whatever price. More needling are the clothes bought on sale that sit in your closet and never get worn. Do the math. If that great "All Sales Final" $50 item bombs when you get it home, it cost you $50 to transport it and you never wore it. If you bought an item for $100, full price, and wore it a hundred times, the cost per wear was $1. That's a bargain!

While you're building your discerning muscle, stick to stores where "sale" items can be returned. Take a pretend truth-finding litmus test and ask yourself honestly if the most appealing quality of the garment on sale is the price tag. The real savings to you may come in walking away.

Clothes Are Like Boyfriends

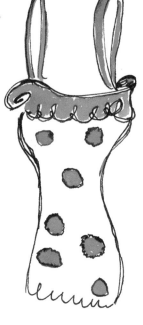

Boy, you sure know how to pick 'em!

~An Anonymous Mom

18

HOW DO YOU PICK A GOOD MAN? Lord knows, there are plenty of ways not to do it, many of which are documented in runaway bestsellers. I believe there are principles women could use to pick a good man (or to walk away from a bad one early on) that also apply to picking out a good, meaningful wardrobe. Or maybe, by learning how to pick out a great wardrobe, you can transfer the how-tos and pick out a good man. Let me know how it turns out.

Review the pitfalls of dating and you'll see there's something to salvage from those bummer dates that will make you brilliant when it comes to clothes. For those of you who got it right, right from the start, you're going to have to use your imagination—like my friend Marie who is out there with no transferable skills whatsoever. At the age of eight, Marie ran away from home and was cooking herself a hot dog in a vacant lot when Carl, who was nine, ambled over, and said, "Whatcha doing?" Well, Carl's father called up Marie's father, who came and took her home, but something sparked and fifteen years later they were engaged, and Carl and Marie have been married ever since.

Others of us have had a few bumps along the road, which is a damn good thing because now we've got a lot of knowledge to apply to the art of getting it right in the clothes department.

You sure know how to pick 'em! Who's fallen for a good label, one that impressed Mom? "He's a doctor, he's a lawyer, he's a CEO." Well, that's nice, but what's he like when you take away the label? I've heard horror stories about boyfriends with great labels but terrible manners, tempers, and drinking problems. It was hard to admit that the guy just didn't work out, because the label was so good and he seemed worth hanging onto.

Likewise, I've seen many a Donna Karan, Armani, or Versace item purchased because of the designer's name, not because of the garment's merit. A label doesn't buy you a foolproof, totally satisfying experience. A woman falls for a Donna Karan assuming the label means it's a good catch, but the neckline that the designer loved that season may not love the purchaser, and it's doomed to sink to the bottom of her closet in uselessness. You have to divorce yourself from the sexiness of the label.

You sure know how to pick 'em! Then there's falling for potential, the fixer-uppers—the jacket that's too long ("I'll move the pockets up and shorten it"), the wrong color ("I'll buy it and dye it"), the hole in the front of the dress that's on sale as is ("I'll just appliqué something right there over the hole, and then I'll appliqué other things over the rest of the dress so it looks like it belongs there"). Recognize a garment's shortcomings early for your peace of mind. You're not going to change that item and make it perfect. Same with the great guy who has his master's degree but doesn't have a job ("I'll help him find work"), spends most of his free time with his buddies in sports bars ("He'll be so in love with me that he'll change"), brags about how he hasn't been out of the county in three years ("He's just not going to the theater, museums, and concerts because he hasn't had a companion as fascinating as I am"). It ain't gonna happen. Move on.

You sure know how to pick 'em! Doesn't it just burn you when you buy the perfect dress, get it home, wear it a couple of times, take it to the cleaners, and it falls apart? It's like the guy who looks dazzling from across the room. He asks you out, you have a lot of laughs over a couple of dinners, and then he totally flakes and your hopes and dreams tumble. That's life. With the guy, you have to move on. With the dress, take it back and complain. Expect to get your money back if you followed the directions for care and it didn't work. A reputable manufacturer will back up their product.

You sure know how to pick 'em! Next, no excuses. Stay alert even while you're falling in love. You know what it's like to fall in love with cashmere. Nothing's come close to touching you like cashmere. You can hardly take your hands off it. You're breathing deeply. Your chest is rising. You're purring. This feeling is, of course, quite wonderful, but it's also dangerous. This is the first sign that you may in fact be losing your mind and unable to see that this very cashmere sweater that's got you drooling all over yourself is orange, a color your skin hates. If a paramedic was nearby, he'd be treating you for assumed food poisoning.

When you're under the spell of cashmere, or the spell of a charming man, you must be willing to ask the hard questions: Does this cashmere sweater (hunky man) really work for me (fit my lifestyle)? Will it hold up over the long haul or is it/he a flash in the pan? Walk away to get out from under the spell and think about it from a different end of town. Face the facts and make no excuses. That gripping love feeling will dissipate and better yet, you'll hold out for the cashmere that's right for you from the start.

You sure know how to pick 'em. Now if you're the kind of woman who can be honest and take responsibility for your actions, you might say, "You know, a rodeo rider may not be long-term relationship material, but, gosh, for a few days in Montana while I'm having some R & R at the ranch, why not?" The zip and zing may be just the thing. Likewise, the trendy velvet animal-print pants clearly aren't going to be the treasure you hand down to your heirs, but it could be great for a fashion fling. Enjoy those tight animal-print pants while they express your folly. Don't measure this by investment or timeless standards, because it isn't in that category. Go forth and play.

You sure know how to pick 'em. If you've been there, done that your whole life, and your closet looks like a costume department for Berkeley Rep, you might be ready to say good-bye to the one-night stands and settle into a long-term relationship with a wardrobe. It's a different mind-set to shop for something that's going to be around for awhile. What should you look for? Start by building a wardrobe around a few colors that you won't get tired of quickly. Consider choosing a couple of your favorite neutral colors—black, brown, navy, gray, olive, taupe, camel, ivory, white. Add splashes of color in smaller things—scarves, blouses. Shop for durable fabrics. A gabardine or a wool/lycra twill will wear for years. A delicate, fine silk georgette will cave in a lot earlier. And remember, those glittery, high-maintenance fabrics aren't always worth the effort required in caring for them. Same with high-maintenance men. Think hard about what you're willing to put up with.

What does this mean when it comes to men? It means you think twice about rock musicians who keep talking about wanting to go on tour. They probably will, which might make having a relationship with him a little more challenging if you're in California and he's in Holland. It also means you give the computer geeks and the guys from the heartland a second look. Don't measure them by Hollywood movie-star standards. They may be just the investment pieces you're looking for—generous, steady, hardworking, committed. It's worth a try.

Good Marriages

Contentment preserves one even from catching a cold. Has a woman who knew she was well-dressed ever caught cold?

~Nietzsche, "Maxims and Missiles"

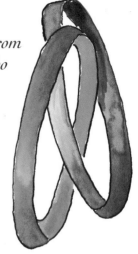

19

DO YOU PUT OUTFITS TOGETHER in the morning, then catch yourself in the office bathroom mirror midday and wonder what the hell's going on here? "What was I thinking?" you ask yourself. Prints are clashing, colors are indifferent to each other, the passion is missing from your ensemble. What went wrong? Has your wardrobe been on the rocks for a long time and you're just noticing it?

You need a little fashion marriage counseling to get everything back on track again. Your prints need to develop better communication skills so they're not screaming at each other all the time. You need to add a little spice to your blah colors, find a way to live with the conflicting opinions of textures. You're in luck. The doctor is in, the remedies are painless. Listen up.

Unless you're wearing a suit everyday, you're putting things together—colors, prints, outfits that include pants, a top, and a jacket—all from different shopping trips. As in a great marriage, the parts are going to come together and create a union that's better than the separates were on their own. Separates are going to live with each other seamlessly like the best marriage you know. Can the Virgo navy pinstripe blazer do the cha-cha with the Gemini floral filmy silk blouse? Maybe Cupid's treated you badly, but in the fashion department, you're about to get lucky.

Fashion Marriage Solution #1: Happily Pairing Prints

Can prints live together? It's a marriage that some people run from, but with a little understanding, you can wear mixed prints confidently. Here's the trick—there needs to be a common color base. Red, white, and blue stars and stripes couldn't hang out with a leafy pattern in rust, olive, and brown. Stay in the same families or tones of a color. A sand, white, and tan floral blouse could be harmonious with a striped scarf in the same colors or tones that are very close. A rust abstract blouse could live with a checked olive and brown jacket because the warm colors are all compatible.

The second thing to consider in pairing prints is scale. They can't be the same scale. One needs to be more dominant. A strong paisley lives happily with a tender check. Bold paisleys and bold checks would fight it out and both would lose. Two prints with equal visual noise, that is, which are both equally active (loud and loud, or quiet and quiet) are doomed. Here's an example of dual prints that work: a multicolored pullover sweater in warm shades with two-inch rows of triangles stacked on top of each other would be content with a pumpkin-colored scarf with a faint olive windowpane check in it. The sweater is louder, the scarf is quieter. Roles are defined. Everybody's content.

Fashion Marriage Solution #2: Creating Harmony While Mixing Colors

Okay, time to solve all color squabbles. If you're a color lover, go for it, but find one way to ground the color group. A good marriage of a black skirt, a lime T-shirt and a coral sweater set would be to let your shoes, belt, and handbag all be black—the rock of the relationship. And if your hair happens to be black, all the better. The eye will start at your shoes and move all the way up your body to your head and create a nice straight line that pulls all the colors together.

This hair trick, matching yours to shoes, belts, and hand-bags, is a good one to follow when marrying separates. Honey-blond leathers for honey-blonds, chocolate-brown leathers for brunettes, black for black and near-black hair colors will con-nect pieces that otherwise would be really unhappy together. Often colors that don't quite match will calm down and get along when you add these accessories. It's like fudging. Close becomes close enough. The eye will move up the body from shoe to belt to hair color and make you look taller and "put together."

If you're wearing a skirt in one color and a top in another, pull the bottom color up to or near your face with a pin that shares the color of the bottom, or an earring or necklace or scarf at the neck that pulls that bottom color up. You'll look much more finished when you're connected.

A print scarf makes a good marriage between two or more solid colors being worn at the same time. Incorporate the clothing colors in the print. If you're wondering whether you can put navy and black together, find those two colors in a print scarf that adds another color or two or three and you'll never step into divorce court.

Fashion Marriage Solution #3: Finding Bliss in Mixed Fabrics

If you love your sturdy wools but are wondering about adding other fabrics to the mix, here's what to do: mix the fabrics in an ensemble while keeping the color the same or of similar tones. Mixing an olive wool slack with a deep moss green charmeuse silk blouse and adding a cashmere cardigan in a deeper olive yet would be luxurious. Add accessories using the same tones or contrast with a belt, shoes, and bag of a rich brown or black. Have you been paying attention? You brunettes or ebony-haired creatures would shine in this outfit.

Fashion Marriage Solution #4: Finding Compatible Lifestyles

Some of you have had trouble with mixed-style marriage — trying to blend your office-life fabrics and colors with your weekend country-flavored togs. You do need to be careful here. Many of your work clothes and play clothes would probably be better left in their own camps, although some key pieces may be flexible enough to live in both worlds. A rich, clean (I mean it doesn't have lots of added details like epaulets or patch pockets) suede jacket could go with your jeans on the weekend as well as with draped trousers, silk blouse, and spiffy leather oxfords for a more dressed-up look. A tweed jacket could be put with slacks and a silk blouse in chocolate brown, or team it with a cotton/lycra white T-shirt and a pair of jeans, boots, and a non-smooth belt in tones matching your hair.

Fashion Marriage Solution #5: Finding Union in Fabric Weights

Caution: A marriage is doomed for divorce court when you try to mix summer-weight fabrics with winter-weight fabrics. I know it's tempting, especially with a dark-colored linen fabric—in black or brown or deep olive. You want to slip it in with wool pieces in November because it goes with your other winter colors. Stop. Linen doesn't belong in your winter wardrobe. It's a hot-weather fabric. Save it for hot weather.

Mazel tov. Best wishes for all your unions. May your wardrobe live the rest of its glorious years in harmony and bliss.

Get Creative, Get Messy

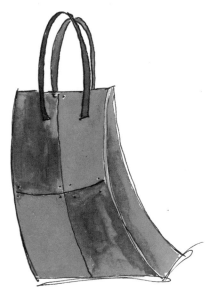

In order to create there must be a dynamic force, and what force is more potent than love?

~Igor Stravinsky, *An Autobiography*

20 THERE'S A PLACE FOR EVERYTHING and everything goes in its place. That might be true and life may, for the most part, actually function better if you put everything back where you found it. But when it comes to creativity and letting the juices have their way with you, you should ignore those military-like rules and regulations and loosen up. Walk into the studio of a revered artist and you'll find paint tubes everywhere, canvasses leaning against every wall. A fiber artist may have her fabrics arranged by color, but when it comes to design, she's got yardage strewn all over the floor or table surface.

And that's what

I'm going to recommend you do to infuse your wardrobe with unexpected delight. Start by throwing your clothes all over your room for a few days in a row. I'm serious. Don't be a neat freak. When everything goes back into your closet neat and tidy day after day, you can get set in your ways. Throwing your clothes all over the room will create wonderful outfits. A purple blouse falling on a cognac skirt may be your next favorite combination. Scarves taken off your neck and tossed onto the pile will resurface with new partners that will thrill you visually.

Sometimes the most delightful sparks can ignite with a little bit of mess. When things are not as they usually are, it jars the mind. You see things differently. Maybe you pick up the black pants off the floor from the day before, grab the curry-colored suit jacket from the back of the chair, and give in to your burning desire to wear pearls. You put them on, turn around, look in the mirror, and it's a hit.

Start a happy riot by mixing up your costume jewelry with your precious jewelry. They'll delight you with new ideas when they're hanging out together instead of being tucked away in some closed drawer.

One of the most creative clothing experiences can be right after a shopping trip. You've been hunting and gathering at the mall, and all the while you're starting to work these pieces into your wardrobe inside your head. Would this lilac blouse on the rack work with your textured linen suit at home? Would the olive shade in this brooch enhance the plain, tailored suit in your closet? Would these black pants in the store be dressy enough for the fuchsia blouse with the covered buttons at home?

You can't wait to see if your outfits will work out in real life the way you've pictured them in your mind. You take your shopping bags up to your room, dump them out on the bed, and start pulling things from your closet. Soon you have blouses and T-shirts on and off, trying them on with your jackets and pants. You go through the whole look from head to toe, trying on jewelry, belts, shoes, and hose, mixing in the old with the new. **This is the time to go for it. The juices are flowing. This could be the most creative few hours you spend all season with your new and old wardrobe, coming up with all kinds of new, exciting outfits.** Stay up late playing with your clothes. You can catch up on sleep another day.

Don't trust your brilliant late-night work to your memory. Those fabulous combos could be forgotten during your sleep as easily as a dream. Use that great journal a friend bought you as a gift that seemed too nice to record your end-of-the-day drivel in. Make it your wardrobe journal and record all the outstanding outfits you've just created. You can also set up a file box using note cards to record your finds. Or, on an 8½" by 11" piece of paper, create a "wardrobe card" that clusters outfits which share pants or a skirt. Choose one bottom piece, a skirt or pants, and write it in a box at the top of the card. Then list all the outfits that can be created with that skirt or pants, including accessories. Put your wardrobe card sheets in sleeve protectors in a three-ring binder. Divide the binder up by seasons or by colors, and refer to it on days when you're not feeling so creative. Or if writing isn't your style, you're more visual, get out your camera and take pictures of each complete outfit, laying them out on your bed including all the accessories. Develop the film, buy a scrapbook to keep the photos in, and keep the scrapbook in a drawer next to your closet so you can refer to it easily.

Another prime creative time to play with your clothes is on the cusp of a season change. Take a look at your summer clothes while there's still a chill in the air. Pull everything out of your closet, try everything on, and see what excites you this year. Be an artist. Having your clothing, your shoes, belts, jewelry, and handbags all around you as materials will inspire you to create art on a new canvas—your body. What pleases you? Start with the piece you're craziest about— a shawl, a favorite pair of shoes—and discover all the new ways of putting outfits together to showcase that item. Your senses will be delighted. It's amazing how a different blouse can revitalize a jacket you've had in your closet for years, which in turn can revitalize your whole week.

Accessories Go to the Movies

My clothes keep my various selves buttoned up together, and enable all these otherwise irreconcilable aggregates of psychological phenomena to pass themselves off as one person.

~LOGAN PEARSALL SMITH, *MORE TRIVIA*

BELIEVE ME, I've heard accessory stories that you wouldn't believe. Neurosurgeons who can connect the tiniest blood vessels freak out when I put a scarf in their hand. "Aaugh, I don't know what to do with this!" they shriek. Accessory Terror! That's what they say, Accessory Terror, which sounds like the name of a movie playing down at the Cinemax.

Well, almost. Anyway, a good movie is what you need to study in order to have the confidence of an award-winning actress when it comes to wearing accessories. You don't need to have a flair, you don't need to be gifted from birth, you don't need to have had a mother who lived for accessories. Just a little understanding will make you a pro.

I don't know if you've seen a good one lately, but a movie

that wins your favor is pulled off with a team effort—a good story, a good director, a great set, superb acting. When you see a woman who you'd describe as being really pulled together and looking sharp, she has assembled her clothes and accessories into a harmonious expression that sends a strong, good message about her.

Let me break it down. If you studied that woman, you might find that her clothing is pretty average, moderately priced, but it's the accessories that have really pulled you in. Her handbag and her shoes are top quality, her watch relates to the mood of her clothing, her earrings and bracelet have a similar theme, and her scarf resting casually around her neck brings her face into focus. Nothing screams "out-of-place." Everything works. It's balanced, and you can't help but enjoy the view.

Look at the art of accessorizing as the art of moviemaking. You're the director of this movie that's you. Your clothes are the scenery or backdrop. Your accessories are the stars in this movie. They are here to help tell the story about you. As the director, you know how temperamental stars can be. The most important thing to remember is to give one accessory top billing. Let one accessory be the star of the show—a luscious scarf that you paid a million bucks for, a wonderful pin you bought at an art gallery, your grandmother's antique cameo brooch. Instruct all other accessories that you're going to wear to "keep it down," take supporting roles, and let the star get the bulk of the attention.

Good supporting actors in a movie are doing their part in the background, but they are integral to the picture. It's the same with supporting accessories. How to do this? Team simple earrings with that antique came brooch. If the brooch is outlined in a shiny, untextured gold, pick up that element, and choose earrings in the same shiny, untextured gold that will support, but not overpower, the brooch. Keep the earrings within the same scale as the brooch. Something big and chunky would grab attention and the brooch would be overlooked. Not good. Kind of like Bronson Pinchot in the 1984 movie *Beverly Hills Cop*. He has a scene with Eddie Murphy, the star with top-billing, who plays the cop. Pinchot plays a jewelry shopkeeper with a goofy accent, and his scene is so funny, so memorable that it won him his own TV sitcom! That's the scene everyone talked about in the reviews and in the neighborhood coffee shops. As entertaining and pleasurable as it was, it broke the momentum of the movie and drew attention to itself.

A good movie is seamless. It creates an overall consistent, believable effect rather than drawing conspicuous attention to any one person or part. Make this your goal in assembling your accessories.

If you're wearing that dynamite scarf your husband bought you on his ski trip, be sure it's the center of attention. Let's say it's made of cut velvet and has an abstract design. The colors are royal blue, deep forest green, and deep fuchsia in a black background. Starting from the feet and moving up, consider black suede shoes, which will support the velvet in the scarf, and a black suede belt at the waist of a skirt or trousers, which keeps the eye moving up the body in a common thread. You might want to pick up a color from the scarf and repeat it in your earrings. You could wear lapis blue earrings rimmed in gold and add a gold bangle at your wrist that repeats the gold to maintain harmony. Don't even think of wearing a sports watch with this ensemble! Keep it simple and elegant, for example, a watch with a gold or a black band.

The biggest mistake in accessorizing an outfit is getting too many disparate elements in there. Everything needs to relate. Just like it does in the movies. When you see a western, you expect to see horses, cowboy boots, cowboy hats, corsets under long dresses with full skirts and crinolines, and a saloon. There wouldn't be a motorcycle, a diner, or beat poets at a poetry reading in North Beach in San Francisco.

If you're a romantic and love lace, antique jewelry, and granny-type lace-up boots, you've got yourself a romance movie right there. All the accessories relate to one another, helping to create that clear theme. As accessories, another romantic movie theme could include a lace handkerchief in a pocket, an antique watch, a pearl necklace, pearl earrings, a long chain with old charms hanging from it, a crocheted hat with a silk flower, crocheted gloves, a small tapestry handbag with a dull-colored gold-link chain (looks old and lovingly worn).

If arty and whimsy is your thing, then your accessories would have that quality.

Perhaps you collect arty pins by clever craftsmen, enjoy novelty watches with cartoon characters, or wear shoes with big colorful bows on them.

A dramatic woman might like strong, contemporary pieces—a memorable bold gold necklace that she'd team with a wide metal cuff on her wrist, strong leather shoes with a modern design, a leather handbag or tote that she wears on her shoulder which is the same color and material as her shoes.

A classic woman might prefer understated accessories, precious jewelry with simple chiffon scarves, classic pumps—nothing too bold or attention getting.

What's your movie theme? Make your life simple by honoring your preference and your favorite expressions, then invest in accessories that work together. If you have a great necklace you're working with, identify good supporting earrings and shop for them. Accessories that relate well together can be teamed over and over again with your various outfits. Then you'll be the leading lady, the one about whom others say, "Gosh, she's so pulled together. I don't know what it is, but she looks great!"

A Scarf Is a Very Useful Thing

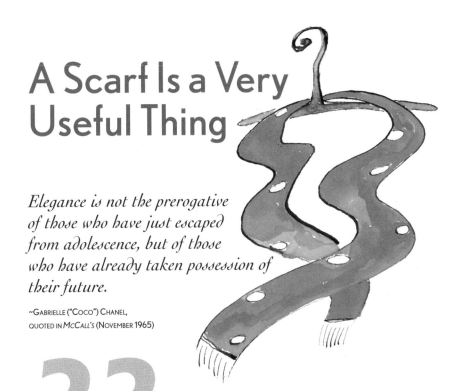

Elegance is not the prerogative of those who have just escaped from adolescence, but of those who have already taken possession of their future.

~GABRIELLE ("COCO") CHANEL,
QUOTED IN *McCALL'S* (NOVEMBER 1965)

22

THE FRENCH WOMAN KNOWS that a scarf is more valuable than rent money. It's hard to believe that across a mere ocean is a land of women in terror of them. How can that be?

Maybe it's the bad rap scarves have gotten in movies.

Let's clear this up right away. As far as I know, only one person has actually died from wearing a scarf and that was Isadora Duncan, the dancer. In the final scene of *Isadora*, starring Vanessa Redgrave as Isadora, she's riding carefree and drunk in an open Bugatti sports car, when the ends of her long red scarf wrap around a gleaming spoked wheel and she's strangled instantly.

And, of course, if you rent *Basic Instinct*, you'll see in the opening scene that an Hermes scarf is an accessory to a violent crime involving an ice pick. That's really too bad. Scarves shouldn't get a bad wrap like that. They are benevolent by nature and only dangerous in the wrong hands. Consider these wonderful things that only scarves can do:

1. They can keep the neck warm as fall leaves fly and winter beckons. Traditional Chinese doctors will advise keeping the neck covered to keep external pernicious influences, especially the wind, from entering the body in the back of the neck. The scarf is preventive medicine.

2. A scarf can contribute to the longevity of suit jackets and blazers by protecting the neckline when worn inside along the collar. Scarves save money that would've been spent at the dry cleaners.

3. Two scarves packed in a suitcase provide variety and entertainment to travel outfits in neutral colors like black, navy, or camel. Tie a scarf to the handle of your generic black suitcase and spot it instantly on the luggage carousel at the airport.

4. A scarf is good for hiding salad dressing tracks on a silk blouse.

5. In the hands of a romantic, a scarf can be a creative tool in the bedroom.

6. A scarf framing a woman's face in luscious colors can give her more confidence, intrigue, and allure than a doctorate degree from Yale.

I doubt the instructional videos in scarf departments in large retail stores inspire anyone. They're boring and dorky. What you need to do is rent some videos on Saturday night with show-stopping scarf scenes.

Start with *Where Sleeping Dogs Lie*, a movie starring Sharon Stone and Dylan McDermott. The first time we see Sharon, she's headed for her white convertible wearing a white (probably Chanel) suit, a white baubley bracelet, and a long white chiffon scarf that trails down her back. It's unlikely that many will wear this look for day, but it sure works for evening, and it's easy. She drives away with the top down, but the windows are rolled up. She's seen the movie *Isadora*.

In *An Affair to Remember*, Deborah Kerr works a similar look. She wears a lovely white ensemble—a sheath dress and matching white coat, white gloves, and a white chiffon scarf floating away from her hair as sheer as a jellyfish—while she slaps a quick, witty, brilliant remark on Cary Grant that leaves him speechless.

The Best Scarf in a Motion Picture appears at the end of *Bodyguard*. Whitney Houston and her entourage are in her private plane and are about to take off when she orders the pilot to stop. Whitney descends from the plane and runs across the tarmac into Kevin Costner's arms. The camera spots the black and white snakeprint scarf that's wrapped around her head and spins around from overhead, showing it from every angle with the theme song welling in the background: "And I-I-I will always love you-ou-ou."

Your scene shouldn't be without a scarf.

Maybe you bought a ladylike fitted suit last month. Line the inside of it with a scarf like Fionna does in the scene from *Four Weddings and a Funeral,* where Hugh Grant ends up at the table with all his past girlfriends.

Maybe you have a short plum-colored knit jumper and you plan to wear a lime green shirt under it. A scarf mixing these colors will add dash to your outfit. Need to see it? Check out Uma Thurman in *The Truth about Cats and Dogs* where Uma's character, as brainy as a bag of nails, is sharp enough to don a kicky neck scarf for a bohemian look that also keeps viral riff-raff out. Two thumbs up.

The Better to See You With, My Dear

Sometimes the eye gets so accustomed that if you don't have a change, you're bored. It's the same with fashion, you know. And that, I suppose, is what style is about.

~BILL BLASS, QUOTED IN *W* (FEBRUARY 1983)

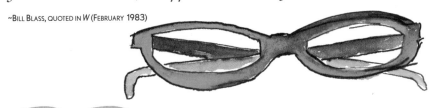

IF YOU WEAR GLASSES, you're potentially way ahead in the style game. You have a reason, a purpose, in fact it's downright necessary for you to wear an accessory on your face. Those of us who are out of luck with near-perfect or 20/20 vision have to work harder at finding a place to leave our mark—or we can fake it! There's nothing like a pair of glasses to add mystery, distinction, style. Think of Jackie Kennedy Onassis, Audrey Hepburn, Sophia Loren. Glasses were integral to their style.

Maybe you're a part-timer. Reading glasses become a sudden necessity in your forties. Don't fight it! Don't hide it! Use it as an opportunity to create a signature. Since "readers" can be very inexpensive when you buy them from a drugstore chain, indulge in several styles—one for every mood—from the quirky reader in you to the studious one. Experiment. Then step up to the next price ranges. You'll find readers at the sunglass counter at department stores. You can also go to an optical store and pick out frames there.

For you full-timers, you must, you must, you must keep updating your glasses. Old styles make you look old, outdated, and tired. They trap you in the decade you bought them in. Shiny silver or shiny gold on the face makes you look older. Look for lenses that pick up your coloring—tones of your hair, eyes, or skin—burnished olive, non-shiny metals, tortoise (both light and dark tortoise), brown, tan, and red. They will be much more flattering to your face. If you've let your hair go gray, try a charcoal frame. It'll bring out the gray, but it won't be harsh like shiny silver would be.

Technology in optics has soared. If you've been slumping behind big thick glasses, you're in for a rebirth. There is nothing to stop you from wearing a modern stylish frame. You can have a progressive bifocal put into a small, thin frame and not only look better but also see better. A smaller lens helps you use the prescription to its full potential.

Frame designs are dramatically updated every two years. When you're at the movies, check out the frames being worn by the stars on the screen. They're usually on the cusp of fashion forward designs. Just observing what they're doing may give you ideas or at least prepare you for the shift in design so it won't seem so different. Sometimes the eye needs a little practice to get used to something new. If you've been paying attention, you're ahead of the game.

Glasses are essential for many people. I want you to think about having an eyeglass wardrobe. I know it's an expense, but you wear these on your face every day. They are extremely important. Consider having a pair for everyday, plus a backup. Then add a dressy pair if you go to a lot of formal functions. This frame can be more ornate, more intriguing and interesting, shinier, more like jewelry.

If you're wearing glasses for your job, you need a pair that optimizes the messages you want to project to those you serve. If you're in a conservative field, you'll stick to classic shapes — circles, squares, ovals, rectangles. Choose a shape that will flatter your features — following the line of your eyebrow, an upsweep style puts the focus right on your eyes, for instance. And don't walk out of the optical office until you've asked for the nonglare protective coating. This cuts the glare, is great for night driving, and is especially important because it lets your audience see your eyes clearly — almost as if the glass wasn't there at all.

If you're in sales or have close contact with people, don't select eyewear that obscures you. If you choose a bright-colored frame, that's all somebody's going to be thinking about when they're looking at you, not about what you have to say. If you're a therapist, you don't want a heavy look in a frame. Go for what looks the most open and nonthreatening. This helps create a sense of safety and openness for your clients. If you've chosen eyewear that is synonymous with your profession, it automatically helps people trust you.

Now where's your fun pair? Your dating pair? Your weekend pair? Frames can express all aspects of you. What should you look for in sunglasses? This is a great place to go big, go glamorous. In a larger frame, more of the area around your eye is being protected. Crow's feet are happiest being in the shade.

Because there's a lot at stake in choosing eyewear, go to a reputable office or boutique. A fast-frame place is not going to have the same interest and expertise in fitting you in the absolute best frame for your personality, profession, and physical features. Make a budget category for eyewear. Glasses speak louder than your voice and even when you don't get a chance to talk to that person across the room, they'll see you and how you look will create a lasting impression. Make it good.

Besides insisting on the nonglare coating, we'll see you better when you go a little bit heavier with your eye makeup. Use a darker liner on the top lid and then go down a few shades and line the bottom lid. This will make your eyes more visible. **And always, always, keep your eyebrow line visible and important.** Keep those brows defined and well-manicured. With that extra action at your eyes, it's important to put your lips on your face map. If your frame is light, keep the lips light. If you're in a darker frame, don't be afraid of color for your lips. The total package makes it all the better to see you with, my dear.

Alternatives to Plastic Surgery

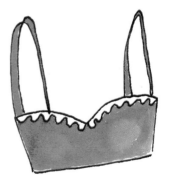

I have never known a really chic woman whose appearance was not, in large part, an outward reflection of the inner self.

~MAINBOCHER, QUOTED IN *VOGUE* (APRIL 1964)

2 4 MY STOMACH REMEMBERS it like it was yesterday's lunch—bad seafood. I was going to Good Guys Electronic Store to buy an answering machine for my kids the afternoon that Phil Donahue was showing an actual face-lift procedure on his award-winning talk show. On all 250 television sets that created three floor-to-ceiling walls, a surgeon had a face splayed open. I recognized an ear. Everything else was quivery, watery, and bloody. He was a leading plastic surgeon from Los Angeles giving blow-by-blow account in close-up shots that never let up.

"Uhh, I'd like to get an answering machine—and do you have a barf bag under the counter?" I asked the nearest salesman. The quivery, bloody close-up shots stayed on the screen the whole time I was in there. They didn't even break for commercials!

Thinking at the time that I didn't wish that procedure on anyone, I became motivated to do everything I could to create sound alternatives for women — and if not to create alternatives, then at least to make the effects of aging more painless. Now I'm not saying never have plastic surgery. Never say never. Not even to blue eyeshadow. You don't know what you're capable of doing ten years from now.

You may be thinking about this already. You may have a bank account set up for surgery. I'm not going to stop you, but I am going to show you some things you can do right now that will give you more lift than you knew possible.

One of the goals of a face-lift is to counter the force of gravity. What goes down, must come up. Eyelids, foreheads, cheeks. Draw it up and tuck it behind the ears and at the hairline at the top of your head. Without spending $10,000, you can create a lot of lift by knowing how to place accessories on and around your face. Consider this: a scarf knotted too low draws the eye down, not up. Experiment with this in front of a mirror. If you're wearing an oblong scarf and it's knotted below your bustline, chances are your audience's attention is not getting to your face very fast. Place that knot between your bustline and your shoulder blades and the attention quickly moves up to the face. Why droop when you can lift? You'll look younger and taller.

An earring should draw your audience's eye up to your own eye quickly. When you're trying on earrings, look in the mirror to see which ones move you quickly to your eyes. Try several pairs on. Watch for speed. The earrings that move your attention to your eyes the quickest deserve a purchase over the slowpokes.

They are working with gravity and you are looking younger.

Some earrings sit too low on the ear and focus attention somewhere down at the middle of your neck. These are drawing the audience's eye down instead of up.

Earlobes that once held a neat, tiny pierced hole, but whose hole is now a ½" vertical line heading south, will also draw the eye down and make you look older. These can be surgically corrected, or you can get a hole pierced above that line if your lobe is big enough and wear earrings that cover it up. You would have to avoid earrings that hang off a wire.

Eyebrows that are not shaped or filled in will make your face drop. The quickest "lift" can come from working on those eyebrows. Often brows thin out as we age, or they might have been altered in our twenties and never recovered. Have your eyebrows professionally shaped and use an angle brush and an eye powder color close to your own, or use an eyebrow pencil to fill your brows in.

When wearing a pin on a jacket lapel, pay attention to the placement. Line part of the pin up with the outer edge of your face or hair. Once again your audience's eye will jump quickly to your face because you're creating a relationship between that pin and your face. A pin that hangs out at the edge of a shoulder, far away from your features, looks like it's trying to get away from you. It's distracting. And don't let it droop down to your bustline. Bring the pin closer to your chin than your bustline to keep the attention moving up to your face instead of dropping to the floor.

Get your hair styled so there's emphasis near eye level. A great cut that highlights your eyes with bangs or waves or that has angles which naturally draw your audience's eyes up to your eyes will make another big shift in perception. You can also have your hairdresser put in highlights that create more light around your eyes.

If you wear glasses, take a look in the mirror. Is the focus on your eyes, or is it on your cheeks? Go to a retail eyeglass store and try on a bunch of frames. Again, you want the attention to zoom up to your eyes. Many of those large frames that people wore in the '80s focused attention on their mid-to-lower cheek and not on their eyes. Wear frames that lift your attention up to your eyes.

Following one or two of my suggestions will help lift up what gravity has dropped. Pay attention to all of these details — the eyebrows, the haircut, the placement of earrings, pins, and scarves—and you'll see a dramatic difference. You will look younger and healthier, which, let's face it, makes us feel better. We're not changing the facts on our driver's license—well, maybe the weight part, but not our birthdate. We are taking advantage of easy tools that will make gravity less of an issue. And it's legal and cheap. Take these steps and live with them for a while. Then take another look at whether you're going to have surgery or not.

Learn a Thing or Two from Men

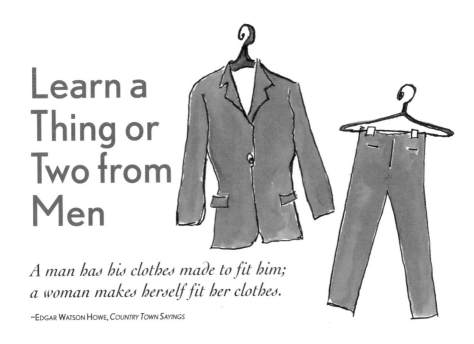

A man has his clothes made to fit him;
a woman makes herself fit her clothes.

~Edgar Watson Howe, *Country Town Sayings*

25

Casual Friday aside; it has been simple for men. Hey, what's simpler than a suit? If you're someone who wants a nice simple recipe for dressing, duplicate what's worked for decades. The brilliance of a suit is this—it's a no-brainer. A matching skirt and jacket or pants and a jacket even in casual fabrics looks instantly put together and smart. It's easy to manipulate a suit's message. The more you want to be taken seriously, the less pattern you want in your suit, and the darker you'll go in color. Fine, tight weaves say "authority," while loose, nubby weaves say "friendly."

Men may select a limited spectrum of shirt colors to wear with their suits, but this is a place where a woman can let 'er rip. Make a color statement. Make that suit snap, crackle, and pop. Put eggplant under an olive suit, persimmon under camel, lime under black, watermelon under charcoal gray.

If you're going to leave mixing and matching to your sister-in-law and wear a suit, then do what every man does—insist on great tailoring, fit that is perfection. Go hang out in a men's suit department and watch the wizard tailors mark a suit with chalk—taking in here, letting out there, lifting this and dropping that. Men expect a lot of things from life that women don't even consider. It's a given for a man to have new clothes tailored to fit him. A woman tries on clothes, expects them to fit her, and when they don't, she thinks something's wrong with the outfit, or more likely, something's wrong with her body that it's not fitting right. Men never make their bodies wrong.

In that same scene in the fitting room in the men's department, he's in a suit that doesn't fit him right. Not yet. But it will. Before you give up or turn away from a great suit, try different sizes. You may go up a size to get it to fit your hips and now it's loose in the waist. Great. Now bring in the tailor. Alterations are a good thing. Insist on them. You'll feel special having your specific body acknowledged and honored with the right fit.

Buy great-looking belts in the men's department. They are often of better quality and have more interesting textures while being less expensive than belts in the women's department. Many belt departments will cut the size down for you for no charge. Or take it to your favorite shoe repair person. You want the belt to fit you comfortably with the notch resting in the third hole of a five hole belt.

Looking for a great scarf to wear inside your winter coat or outside your suede jacket with jeans and boots on a crisp fall day? Hike those pointy-toed Manola Blahniks of yours down to a great men's furnishings department. (Furnishing: 1. A piece of equipment necessary or useful for comfort or convenience. 2. furnishings. Wearing apparel and accessories.) They know just what comfort is there. You'll find lush chenilles, the softest wool plaids, prints that look like modern art museum paintings, great color mixes, great fabrics. Menswear is famous for their fabrics and gazillion variations on a pattern. Go where the experts are and show some originality in your furnishings.

A man expects his clothes will stick around awhile. He'll put out the bucks for quality. He's seen what happens to that suit with the fused lining after a few cleanings versus the suit with the hand-stitched inside construction that helps the suit hold its shape for years. **Buy quality for those pieces you want hanging around for a long time.**

Keep your shoes shined. When your shoes look haggard, so do you. For a $3 investment at the shoe repair shop on the corner, they will look like new and so will you.

And lastly, don't wimp out at the cash register. If you put together a wardrobe for a man, he thinks you're brilliant and will whip out the credit card and not edit a thing. A woman filters her purchases through her "Am-I-Worth-It" lens and loses her nerve at the cash register. Come on, girls! You're worth that and more! Throw your shoulders back, stand tall, and please yourself. **Put yourself top on the list.**

Be selfish. It's all good.

Friendly
Forgiving Fabrics

*I always wear slacks because of the brambles
and maybe the snakes. And see this basket?
I keep everything in it. So I look ghastly, do
I? I don't care — so long as I'm comfortable.*

~KATHERINE HEPBURN, QUOTED IN
KATE BY CHARLES HIGHAM

26

BACK IN OUR TWENTIES, fabric decisions were
easy. We were card carriers of the natural
fibers club. If it wasn't a fabric made out of
cotton, linen, wool or silk, it was bad for you. Everybody knew
that polyester was for retirees, car salesmen in Butte who
smoked cigars and told trashy jokes, or tourists flocking to San
Francisco's Fisherman's Wharf in February. Our mothers fell
under the spell of polyester because it let them put away their
ironing boards for good. Daughters were aghast. How could
mothers not see that polyester was bad for you? Spray starch,
spray water-bottles, and irons were but a small price to pay for
wearing natural fiber fabrics.

While we were cringing at the sight of man-made polyester,

most of us weren't aware of all the chemical processes that natural fiber fabric goes through before it gets on our backs—dying as well as cleaning and repairing processes. The softer the fabric, the more chemical processes it's been through. Burlap, now that's the closest we might come to a "natural" natural fabric—but do you want to wear it?

To be a stickler today and insist on 100 percent natural fibers is like saying, "Thanks very much, but I'm sticking to this manual typewriter that I can't buy ribbons for. Computers are not for me." Those chemical companies actually have your best interests in mind. Really.

Technological advances in fabric move forward faster than our birthdays. And being the environmentally aware gang that we are, it's refreshing to discover that even those two-liter Coke bottles are being recycled into fabrics. If you wear a cuddly, warm polartec fleece fabric in a casual jacket, its past life was as a shelf-full of plastic Coke bottles.

Wearing polyester in the '70s was like wearing a plastic bag. Now polyester fibers are fine and strong, and they allow breathability. They feel more natural than natural fibers, and often hold up to stain and wear better.

One of my favorite polyester fabrics is microfiber. It's silky, breathable, smooth, velvety, drapes beautifully, and is water repellent. Each strand is 1/100 the size of a human hair. That dense weave is what makes it so darn nice to touch, yet it's tough as nails—you can't put a pin through it. When water hits the surface, it beads up and falls off, defenseless, making it perfect for raincoats, casual jackets, shoes and boots, and handbags. It is much lighter weight than leather so shoe, handbag, and coat manufacturers are using it in their high fashion designs, sometimes adding leather trim as accent. Technology is your friend, girlfriends. Now apologize to your mom for being such a non-know-it-all, after all.

Technology is also on your side if you're active in sports. Cotton is rotten for the athlete because it holds water when you sweat. If it's colder outside than your body is, perspiration cools down while evaporating and you can get hypothermia. You want moisture to move away from the skin during those wild bike rides, intense runs, or fierce roller derby matches. This is possible with the new fabrics that wick the moisture away from your body. The next best fabric to choose for sports is wool, which keeps you warm in the winter and cool in the summer.

Having workout clothes that provide these kinds of benefits will keep you in the sport longer. You advance in a sport more quickly if you do the small things that make a big difference, starting with dressing for comfort.

The best place to discover the latest in new fabrics and new fabric treatments is in the activewear departments, where new fibers are tested because of the lower price points (clothes with lower price tags). If a fabric does well there, it'll move up the fashion food chain into day wear, then business wear, and finally into evening wear.

Think back on Lycra. You probably first bought it in leggings and leotards, and now you find it in everything. Lycra is your friend. A little of it (2–4 percent) will give a fabric memory, which means fewer wrinkles, more smoothness (we all can use some more smoothness past forty), and more durability. Suits with Lycra blended into the fabric give two-way stretch, making movement easier in the shoulders and arms. Clothes can fit closer to the body because of the ease that Lycra provides. Other fabrics would strain, pull, or split at the seams. Lycra is added to wool, silk, cotton, and now linen, which, if you're wrinkle phobic, cuts the amount of wrinkles.

Do you need the
perfect body to wear close-fitting clothes?

Not with Lycra in the blend. You may want to go up a size so the clothes don't feel too snug, but please, don't be afraid of a silhouette. The fabric may create new possibilities for shapes that you never wore before.

Fabrics that have some drape to them—a crepe, jersey, tencel—grace the body sensually and are preferable for curvy bodies that need a fabric to gently drape over those curves. Fabric with "body" will stand away from the body and not cling or expose rolls.

Thick fabrics add bulk. Fabrics that are thin or have drape remove bulk. Nancy Reagan wore bouclé suits. She was a tiny little thing and adding bulk worked for her. I wouldn't recommend it for Barbara Bush, who would look like a kid stuffed inside a zipped-up snowsuit in a North Dakota blizzard.

If you come across a challenging label with words you can't read or understand, ask a salesperson if they've had experience with this fabric. Has anyone returned an item for poor performance? If not, pay close attention to the care instructions and follow them. The manufacturer has done its best to figure out the care of these wild blends, and sometimes they get it wrong. If the garment doesn't hold up, return it and get your money back.

Fit, Fat, or Fake It

I think self-awareness is probably the most important thing towards being a champion.

~Billie Jean King, quoted by Marlene Jensen in *The Sportswoman* (November/December 1973)

SEE IF YOU CAN RELATE. It happens every summer around bathing suit time. I think of doing something about these extra five pounds, the five on top of the other five that I've made friends with. Magazines on the racks at the grocery store checkout line shout in bold, red, cheerleader print: Lose 10 Pounds in 10 Days. I don't think so.

I consider counting fat grams, but it's peach season. Can I help it if I make the best peach pie this side of Billings, Montana? I've thought of topping it off with nonfat frozen yogurt instead of Ben and Jerry's Vanilla Mega-Fat Ice Cream

—until I tried it. It doesn't work.

I could bounce out of bed every morning and hit the trails —except that I bought new sheets. I wake up every morning and I'm in a sea of summer flowers—irises, old-fashioned roses in white and pink, blue bells touching my toes. It makes more sense, somehow, to enjoy nature right here in bed.

I could always break up with my boyfriend. That would be good for five or six pounds. He's a pretty sweet guy though. He wears contact lenses that he takes out every night before going to bed. His world gets all fuzzy. I like that in a guy.

There's got to be an easier, softer way.

The solution is right in front of me. I can follow my own fashion advice! There are faster ways to lose weight, at least visually, without diet or exercise. I'm busy. For right now, I'm just as happy looking thinner as being thinner. I'll lose ten pounds in ten minutes, my way.

Staring into the mirror, I can see that I'm still my basic shape, just a little thicker—expect for my eyebrows. They're thinner. I can fill them in with strokes of Blonde Beauty eyebrow pencil and the focus will shift up to my peaches-and-cream complexion where I welcome the attention.

I move down to my shoulders. New York designers may be arguing about whether to pad or not to pad, but I know that even a smallish pad makes my shoulders broader than my hips. That's good for four pounds. The stationary bike stays in storage.

Next, the bustline. Looking in the mirror I can see that my bustline does not sit right in the middle anymore between my shoulder line and my waistline. There's been a slippage of two or three inches. A low bustline makes women look heavier than they actually are. By adjusting my bra straps I work that line back up toward the middle. I practically look perky. Minus three pounds.

Next, my waistline. Belts pulled tight make the tummy protrude. Tighter never looks thinner. It looks fatter. By loosening the belt a notch or two, making it look relaxed, I've lost a pound or more. This is easier than making pie crust.

With two pounds to go, I tackle pants. Clothes too tight (as in a seam that pulls, a pleat that splits open rather than lays flat) add more pounds, even on thin people. Wearing a size bigger can make you look a size smaller. I'm prepared.

It seemed so hard mentally to go up a size until I saw the results. I was at the Gap with my teenaged daughter, joined her in the dressing room and tried on a size 12 for the first time. They fit with room to spare. My daughter said, "Looks great, Mom. Buy 'em."

So that's how I came to have a larger pair of jeans in my closet, which is a good thing. I got on a scale this morning, something I do as often as cleaning skylights, and it read 145. I've never seen that number before except in my checkbook register. I took drastic measures. I said, "So what?" I filled in my brows, adjusted my bra straps, slipped in my shoulder pads, pulled on my new jeans, loosened my belt, and got on with life.

I met my friend Marie for lunch. We argued while eating vegetables and rice in green coconut sauce. She insisted I'd lost weight. I said I hadn't. She waved her eggroll at me, "Yes, you have. I know you have." I said, "Okay, okay, I've lost ten pounds. Buy me dessert and I'll tell you how I did it."

Dressing for Your High School Reunion

*The apparel oft proclaims
the man.*

~SHAKESPEARE, *HAMLET*

28

THE INVITATION COMES in the mail with a postmark from the past. "Fellow classmate," it reads, "Our high school reunion wouldn't be complete without you there." Visions of Robert Frank, Susie Shelby, and Kathy Martin flood your head. You write the check, lick the envelope, wonder if Roger Ellison ever got out of jail, and drop your registration in the mail. You have only six weeks to obsess over what you're going to wear. You know people will be cramming before this event. They'll be poring over yearbook pictures, trying to memorize faces. Be smart. Don't wait until the last minute. Handle the clothes early on so when the day rolls around you can relax and be "yourself," which you've now had twenty-five years to perfect.

Your face may have been a blur in the crowd of protesters

picketing the dress code regulations in front of the principal's office, but now it's time to step out and be noticed. Be memorable that first night by wearing clothing in colors that repeat your own coloring. If you repeat your eye color in a blouse or a dress, you'll hold everyone's attention. There are plenty of subtle variations in blues and greens within fashion choices. You'll have no problem satisfying any hue from those families— true blues, smokey blues, azure blue, and greens from sage to aqua to sea foam. Brown-eyed beauties can go for chocolates or raisin browns for instant recognition.

Go for broke and add your hair color. Wear it in your clothes or in accessories. A rich brown pair of shoes, belt, and handbag will draw your classmate's eyes straight up to your auburn hair. Honey blondes can wear palomino colors, ash blondes can wear taupes beautifully, redheads look glorious in rust or brick, and of course, black-haired women are stunning in black and charcoal. Gray-haired women can wear soft metallics in silver or platinum. A whole column of color, head to toe, that matches one of your own colors is quite impressive. And hey, a high school reunion is exactly where you want to be impressive. It's time to show that guy who dumped you in your sophomore year for Renee Deasdale that he made a tragic mistake.

If you're looking for romance at your high school reunion, wear the soft peaches and pinks that repeat your skin tone. Put those colors in some real touchy fabrics—soft silks, lightweight cashmere, velvet. You'll be irresistible. Women, don't walk out of the house without filling in those eyebrows. They may have faded a bit, and your features will fade out too without this natural frame for your face.

If you are thin enough to be wearing the same size as you wore in high school, you're in big trouble. Besides the fact that you could get sent to the principal's office for that, it could mean you're still wearing those same high school outfits. Look like you've kept up with the times by showing up in current styles.

If you've been fortunate enough to have gained some weight, you're more likely to have bought clothes in recent times. Wearing current clothing styles makes you look youthful.

If you want to camouflage any extra pounds, follow these tips:

1. Don't wear anything that strains the seams of your clothes. Wear a size bigger to look a size smaller. Clothes that effortlessly drape your body make you look prosperous as well. Tight clothes make you look cheap.

2. Wear the same color on the top as you wear on the bottom. All black, all navy, or all plum creates a long vertical line that keeps our eyes moving up and down. This makes you look thinner. And who said you'd never use geometry?

3. If your shoulders are sloping, you'll look heavier than you are. Dumpy, actually. Add a shoulder pad that will straighten out that line. Adding a little definition at the shoulder line takes visual pounds off your hips.

If you were treated like a nerd and never got any respect in high school, try some color psychology on your classmates. Wear navy blue, black, or charcoal gray with stark white. The high contrast of light and dark colors sends an authoritative, don't-mess-with-me message. Crisp fabrics (not wimpy) with fine finishes also add authority to your presence.

If you were the bookworm who graduated with a GPA above a 4.0, you're probably ready to show those clowns that you had a sensual side all along as well. Wear fabrics that drape your body—a liquid matte jersey knit would do the trick. Wear your contacts and show off your shoulders. A cleavage-enhancing bra isn't a bad idea either. Those guys who hounded you will be picking their jaws up off the table.

And here's advice for the girls voted "Least Likely to Make It through High School without Getting Pregnant at Least Once." They never saw you from the waist up, but they will if you wear stiffer fabrics. Nothing clingy. Add a pinstripe to your outfit. Creating a straight up and down detail like that will send more respect your way. Those jerks. All that teasing you had to endure. Adding a police chief for a husband as an accessory on your arm might be a nice touch.

Dressing for Divorce

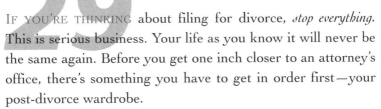

She dressed more severely than was her fashion, needing herringbone for backbone . . .

~DOROTHY SALISBURY DAVIS,
"THE PURPLE IS EVERYTHING"

29

IF YOU'RE THINKING about filing for divorce, *stop everything.* This is serious business. Your life as you know it will never be the same again. Before you get one inch closer to an attorney's office, there's something you have to get in order first—your post-divorce wardrobe.

Your three-hundred-and-fifty-dollar-an-hour lawyers will handle the property settlement, the pension fund, insurance policies, and child support, but do they know anything about clothes? No. They'll say that what's in his closet is his and what's in her closet is hers. The same goes for jewelry and "personal items," which means she gets the tampons and he gets the hair renewal products.

Take it from a 1989 divorce veteran—you'll be losing your

mind by the eighth round of fighting over furniture, family photos, and chipped wooden spoons. Unless you handle it early on,
you'll neglect the only thing that's legally yours anymore—your
personal appearance. Stop filling out the paper-
work for a minute and listen up.

1. Buy new underwear. If he left you for
   another woman, you need new underwear. If you left him for another
   woman, you need new underwear.
   Chances are you need new underwear
   no matter what. What's next to your skin is your
   private pleasure. Take it where you can get it.

2. Destroy your ratty old clothes. You need respect. Ditch the
   stained, faded, ripped clothes you've held onto throughout
   your miserable life together. Those grease-stained sweats
   may have slipped by your lousy husband who didn't notice
   anyway, but they're not good enough for your new life.

3. Stock up on sturdy shoes. Once you file those papers, you'll
   be looking for places to live, employment, and new shoulders to cry on. While you want to be under your favorite
   blankey, sniffing your pillow, there won't be time for rest.
   Hit the pavement with a comfortable shoe—a handsome,
   soft-leathered loafer that caresses your foot with a cush-
   ioned sole that absorbs the shock of uneven pavement.

While you're at it, ditch those four-inch spiky heels he liked
so much. Life is precarious enough without walking around on
pencil sticks. If you're sitting in your closet tossing them back-
ward over your shoulder, watch out that your husband isn't

walking into the room at that very moment. The tips are so pointy they could practically take his eye out. We wouldn't want that now, would we?

4. Dump the stupid presents he gave you. Remember those things he bought you—the skimpy baby doll nighties that you shivered in, the skinny gold chains that were good for nothing, the anniversary blouse he bought in a size too small, on sale—and you hung unto them because you didn't want to hurt his feelings? Dump them. He's going to learn pretty darn quick that you're worth full price.

5. Get rid of that tangled mess of scarves. You've got a drawer full of useless, dinky old scarves. Throw the whole mess out and start fresh. Buy yourself a gorgeous, large silk chiffon scarf, one with substance. Wrap it effortlessly around your neck over any old thing and you'll look gorgeous, whether you're going to the 7-Eleven for milk or Ned's and Ted's for drinks. Your next lover, someone who *really* knows how to make love to a woman, will have his own ideas about what to do with that scarf. Trust me on this.

6. Buy yourself a great belt. Make it an expensive-looking one, so when you lose all that weight during the divorce, you have something really attractive to hold up your pants.

Don't despair. While you're feeling overwhelmed and kicked in the stomach, you'll look like a million bucks. With any luck at all, you'll get through this before your hair falls out.

And remember, without you around to shop for him, he'll soon be looking washed up in clothes he picks out for himself.

Looking great is the best revenge.

Accessorizing
Jammies

*Isn't elegance forgetting what
one is wearing?*

~YVES SAINT LAURENT, *NEW YORK* (NOVEMBER 1983)

30 I GET FRANTIC CALLS every fall when the kids head back to school. Everyone gets their panties in a twist. Like Barbara, Jason's mom, who forgot everything over the summer. It's Wednesday morning, 7:15. Standing under the interrogating glare of the overhead lights at Safeway supermarket, she stares into the dairy case and asks herself this multiple-choice question: Does her fifth grader like custard yogurt, 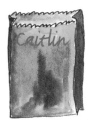 yogurt with granola, or fruit-flavored yogurt in his school lunch? And if it's the fruit-flavored yogurt, which flavor is it? Kiwi? Lemon-Lime? Wild Berry Berry? This is a timed test. She's driving car pool in twenty-five minutes.

She knew it was dangerous not to cram the night before for the School Lunch Test, but there was no way she was going to miss the Emmy Awards on TV. Grownups in dress-up clothes. She needed to review that whole concept. Anyway, she would just get up a little earlier the next morning, hop out of bed, run to the store, and wing it. She'd go in her jammies if she had to. Who would she run into anyway?

Poor thing. She called to tell me she got caught. "Mrs. Rudyan?" a deep voice announced in Aisle 3. It was the vice principal, the one who'd called the day before about her son's language in art class. She was mortified. It's kind of hard standing up for your kid when you're in jammies and beaten-down moccasins that you only use when washing the car.

I told her what I'm telling you: There is a way to look radiant and sharp in jammies. You never have to look sheepish in the checkout line when you follow this advice.

It's best to start with basic two-piece jammies. Nightshirts, ruffles, and pj's with feet in them are tough to work with. A cotton legging and V neck long-sleeved top in heather gray, black, or ivory is a good start. Avoid patterns of cows jumping over moons or happy pigs in polka-dotted dresses. Plain colors in ribbed knits, waffle-knit weaves, or a plain knit weave is good.

Here are the essentials to pull it all together, starting with:

#1: Great Earrings and Lipstick

Put on an attractive pair of earrings, earrings that grab attention, not everyday ones that fade away. Distinctive earrings will throw off the people you run into. You'll look like you're really ready for your day.

Whether you have time to brush your teeth or not, add

color to your face with vivid lipstick tones. It'll brighten your face and give people something to focus on besides the creases on the side of your face from your scrunched-up pillowcase.

#2: $264 Belt (or a strong look-alike)

Thermal jammies look like thermal jammies until you belt them with an expensive, the-real-thing crocodile belt. Maybe you have one hanging around from the '80s. That'll do. Or go buy a pretend one for less money.

If your eyes are brown and the belt is brown, all the better. It keeps our eyes headed up and away from the jammie wrinkles. Hang the belt a little lower than your waist, relaxed, not cinched. Then pull the jammie top over the expensive-looking belt, just a little bit. The slight gathers that creep over the belt make the wrinkles look planned.

#3: Boots and Scrunchy Socks

If you've got brown hair, wear brown boots. If your hair is black, wear black boots. If you're a blond, wear taupe or camel boots. If you have purple hair, you're not worried about running into anybody. Repeating your hair color makes whoever sees you zip from your hair to your boots and back up again, fast, so their eyes don't linger too long on the jammies.

#4: Arty Leather Handbag

You might have picked up a great little hand-crafted shoulder bag at the annual fall festival fair. It adds a lot of class to jammies. Sloppy handbags add nothing. You can have the bag ready at all times, hanging near your closet with a $20 bill and a blank check in it—plus maybe a tube of lipstick, in case you're applying your lipstick in the car while at a stop sign because you didn't have time to do it at home.

#5: Long, Great Coat

A long coat adds a real clean line to jammies. Neatens everything up. Make it a coat with style. It can be slouchy, like a bathrobe really. Relaxed, with interesting pockets, a sturdy collar that can stand up if you like that look. Don't close it. You have nothing to hide, remember? Just let it hang open, loose.

#6: Long, Soft Scarf (optional)

Wrap it oh-so-casually around your neck, Isadora-Duncan-like, only don't do this if you drive a convertible. Isadora's long scarf got locked around the wire wheel of her sports car, and it strangled her. Don't take any risks. If you drive an SUV, or a Volvo station wagon, you can add the scarf for textural interest.

With practice, accessorizing jammies takes only a minute. You'll be able to run into an ex-lover or the town gossip while standing in the checkout line and get nothing but compliments. Like I told Barbara, the toughest part will be when someone says, "Gee, Barb, you look great!" and you're going to want to say, "This old thing? I'm wearing my jammies!" Refrain. Just smile and say, "Thank you."

How to Buy a Bathing Suit

First teach a person to develop to the point of his limitations and then — pff! — break the limitation.

~VIOLA SPOLIN, QUOTED IN
"SPOLIN GAME PLAN FOR IMPROVISATIONAL THEATER"
BY BARRY HYAMS (*LOS ANGELES TIMES*, MAY 26, 1974)

31

BATHING SUIT. I don't know of any other two words put together that scream "terror" quite like BaThInG sUiT.

I was in a dressing room, having selected several bathing suits for my forty-six-year-old client to try on. I was unclipping two-pieces from the hangers as she was slipping out of her clothes. She stopped. Her face went white. Her words came out despite her held breath, "Trying on bathing suits makes me suicidal."

I was cavalier. It was easy for me. I was *not* the one getting naked. Instead of calling 911, ever optimistic, I said, cheerily, "Oh, I think you'll be surprised." But for the first five minutes my stomach was having copycat feelings of dread. Trying on bathing suits is scary, depressing, awful — like getting food poisoning.

The good news is, it got better. Way better. My client left the dressing room forty-five minutes later with a bathing suit wardrobe—two suits and three cover ups ranging from glamorous to sporty. She left the department with a non-medicinally-induced smile on her face. She left with soaring self-esteem.

Impossible, you say? No, this can happen to you too, without the aid of drugs. I promise. Of course, if you're one of the five people in America with a flawless body, you don't need my help. But if you're someone who thinks they have "body considerations" with no access to airbrush equipment, you will be interested in the friendly nature of spandex, prints, texture, and underwires. You see, everything's right about your body. It's just finding a bathing suit that agrees with it. You may have to try on some duds before the prince emerges, but the right bathing suit is out there waiting for you.

Here are some tips for spotting them:

1. You know how sunscreen comes in greater and greater quantities of protection, SPF 2–45? Well, bathing suit fabrics come in greater and greater amounts of spandex, the better to smooth and trim, my dear. Check the label. It could have 31 percent spandex in it. Some suits come with tummy control built into the front panels.

2. Smooth fabrics, especially shiny ones, show the caloric content of lattes, but fabrics with texture will conceal slight bulges and dimples.

3. Pattern, like floral prints on suits, is great for entertaining the eye and inviting it not to rest on any one part of your body that you normally obsess on. In the same manner,

color blocking, which visually pulls the eye in one direction is great for taking the heat off a part of your body that you feel gives you trouble. If you're focused on your thighs, wear a suit that is periwinkle on the top one-third and navy blue on the bottom two-thirds. The eye will focus on the bustline, not on the thighs.

4. If you are big-busted, wear a suit that has wide straps, both for better support and also to balance the proportion of the bustline. Spaghetti straps and a large bust doesn't look as balanced as a wide-strap suit and a large bust.

5. Smaller-busted women are flattered by halter-style suits and underwire tops with subtle padding to shape the bustline.

6. Graphically printed suits can trim a waistline. They can even create the illusion of a waistline that isn't there with seams or panels that are vertical and curving.

7. Mail-order catalogs like J. Crew (1-800-562-0258) and Eddie Bauer (1-800-426-8020) carry two-piece suits that can be ordered in separate sizes, if you're one size on the top and another size on the bottom.

If this is just all too complicated, you have two more choices. First, click into Jantzen's web site (www.jantzenswim.com). Get interactive with suit styles that match your figure concerns before you set foot in a dressing room with trick mirrors designed to spotlight every speck of cellulite. (Remember; without air brushing, models have cellulite too). Or second, say screw it and go splish-splash in whatever you have in your drawer and remember the whole point of donning a suit is to prepare you for

Fun,

Fun,

Fun! Stop fussing and have some.

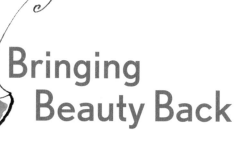

Bringing Beauty Back

I'm tired of all this nonsense about beauty being only skin-deep. That's deep enough. What do you want — an adorable pancreas?

~ JEAN KERR, *THE SNAKE HAS ALL THE LINES*

FIRST OF ALL, you have to know that women tell me everything. When a woman stands in front of a full-length mirror inside a dressing room stripped down to her panties and bra, nothing but truth falls from her lips. Tender vulnerable truth. So believe me when I tell you that every single woman I've met who's in her forties is interested in the same thing. Oh, they might want help finding appropriate casual Friday duds, an interview outfit that shows off their smarts, or clothes for the office that are understated, comfortable, manageable yet authoritative. But for women who powered through the '80s and nested in the '90s, what they want now is to get back to expressing their femininity. Women are wanting to look like women — sensual, sexual, pretty, attractive.

We're not talking bimbo attire here. Not San Francisco Tenderloin district hot pants, push-up bras, fishnet stockings, and spiky heels. Not sexiness for money but sexiness for personal pleasure.

This is not for the purpose of attracting men (even if it's their husband), or if that is a factor, it's secondary. No, this is personal. A college professor says, "I want to honor my sexuality." A business consultant wants to express "grown-up gorgeous." A full-time carpooling mom says, "I want more femininity, even in my jeans and T-shirts."

After years of power dressing or dressing like men, femininity may not be your strong suit, but we'll change that. Start by staying out of your sweats for two weeks. If it looks like gym clothes, keep them at the gym. Let the power suits collect some dust. Put away the armor clothes and pull out the amour clothes. Have a love affair with yourself. Dress for your own scintillating pleasure.

Pick from these ingredients for your own recipe for lusciousness.

Show Some Skin: This can be as subtle as choosing a cotton T-shirt that has a scoop neck instead of a crew neck. Unbutton a couple of top buttons on a blouse. Wear a black camisole under a sheer black blouse or under a flocked velvet blouse. You don't need perfect arms when layering sheer fabrics. Highlight great legs with shorter skirts and textured hose. Wear open-toed shoes or sandals that show off your well-groomed and polished tootsies.

Outline the Body: Lots of garments are made with fabrics that blend in 2–4 percent Lycra or spandex, so they fit closer to the body while still being comfortable when you move and stretch your limbs. If you've been working out at the gym, this won't make you nervous. If not, you may think you can't wear close-fitting clothes. Not true. Bring willingness with you when you shop for the sensual you, because I want you to try on clothes from many different companies—don't give up! You will find both tops and bottoms that grace and define your body without making you feel trashy. Try going up a size or two to get the fit you're comfortable in. If you wear a close-fitting top in jersey or knit, wear a drapier pant for a not-overly-revealing look. Or reverse it and wear close-fitting pants with a lustrous taffeta blouse. Tuck your shirt into your underwear or panty-hose for a smoother line.

Wear Sensual Fabrics: Who can resist velvet? A carpooling mom can wear velvet in a 100 percent washable jean. A long velvet scarf inside a coat can make you feel delicious. Don't save cashmere for good. Wear it every day. Silk charmeuse will make you feel sumptuous. Suede can make you purr. Leathers can be stiff or as soft as butter. Your body will prefer butter leather, believe me. Sexy underwear is a must—even if you work at the post office in a uniform. Especially if you work in a uniform. Whether you're the lacy type or you prefer a silk-satin bra and panty set in black or apricot, make your underwear sizzle.

Next time you're walking through a store, focus on your sense of touch. Touch everything in sight and discover what you like the best. Only wear what you love to touch.

Add Shine: Shine used to be only in evening wear or dress-up clothes. Now it's in "every" wear. A garment with shine, sheen, or luster appears more glamorous and feminine than a dull fabric. If you're wearing shine, try highlighting it by making everything else a matte finish—matte pants and suede shoes with a lustrous blouse. One hit of shine is often enough. Too many pieces of shine in one outfit is distracting.

Bring Focus to the Face: Expose one ear by pulling your hair back. If your hair is long, wear it up with some parts cascading down. Wear earrings that have movement. Make lips look fuller by extending just beyond your lipline with a lip pencil and then filling in with lipstick color.

Be luscious. Be liquid—soft, inviting, touchable. Enjoy the heck out of yourself. The film is rolling and you're the glamorous movie star on the screen. Pamper and practice until you find yourself irresistible. Now that's power dressing!

Where to Get a Clue

*The most evident token and apparent sign of true
wisdom is a constant and unconstrained rejoicing.*

~MONTAIGNE: *ESSAYS*

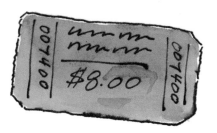

33 IT'S EASY TO BE FORTY or more and think you've been there,
done that, and run out of ideas. Don't tell me you're thinking of
giving up on fashion and style altogether and leaving it for the
teenagers to toss around. No sir-ee, babe! You're still in the
game. There are plenty of moves out there begging to be
enjoyed by your luscious self, and they're destined to generate
pleasure from your hair follicles to your toenails. You're forty,
you've earned the right to do just about anything you damn
well please, so put on your seat belt, we're going for a fun ride.
I'm going to start you out, scratch the surface of ideas, and
before you're done with this, you'll have thought of ten other
things you want to try.

Inspiration comes from lots of places. It comes from the

bundles of daffodils springing up around town that remind you to pull out and wear those bright, spring colors. It's on your TV in the dozens of makeover shows that give you a new idea for your hair. It's in the crosswalk when an especially attractively attired woman walks toward you. It's in the store window you pass on your way to pick up some hosiery; it's in the whimsical, colorful presentation of food at your favorite restaurant. It's at the ballet in the dancers' sequined and beaded costumes.

Good ideas are out there for you, begging to be stolen, manipulated, and presented as original just as they are for fashion designers who have to come up with three to five lines or more a year for their buying public. How do they stay inspired? They travel, like you do. They get ideas in the shower, like you do. They read about history, like you do, and they go to movies, like you do. They people watch, like you do, and then they translate their ideas into clothes a few months later that are worn by models and marched down runways in New York and Europe.

With the remote control in your hand, be a copycat from your couch. Stylists make a living making other people look good for TV. Check the stars out. Keep abreast of style, hair, makeup, and clothing trends by watching hosts of and guests on entertainment shows, such as *Entertainment Tonight*, the *Rosie O'Donnell Show*, *Oprah*, and the late-night shows. Many soap opera characters are dressed in the latest styles and colors and can be studied for ideas.

InStyle magazine offers plenty of ideas on

style. *Mode* magazine, targeted for women in sizes 12, 14, 16+ (all models are plus sizes), demonstrates style, sexiness, playfulness, and intelligence in their fashion spreads featuring women with bodies that reflect America's average rather than the broomstick-shaped teenage models in most fashion magazines.

Read interior decorating or gardening magazines, and look at color and design. Architecture magazines will inspire moods that you can then translate into clothes. Browse through books on art and the history of costume. Good design will leap out at you and beg to be copied.

Go to the movies. Gwyneth Paltrow, in the second half of the movie *Great Expectations*, demonstrates the power of a killer lipstick color (in high contrast to a natural face with barely-there makeup) that perfectly matches or complements her Donna Karan clothes. Rent *Wings of the Dove* if you want to get yourself out of a chino and T-shirt rut. The clothes, vastly rich in detail, will take your breath away with their tucks and gathers, hand embroidery, a zillion teeny buttons on a bodice, and beaded handbags. You'll be inspired to pull out the stops and slip into some deliciously feminine clothing. Often popular flicks can create a fashion flash on their own. Who can forget the Annie Hall look? Make your own flash by translating what you see on the screen into your own style. Pay attention to what pleases you. Looking for style clues makes sitting through an otherwise no-good movie a pleasure. Remember, a lot of money has gone into planning those costumes. It's like drinking scotch straight—nothing's been watered down. Every effort has been made to create believable characters. So the details are there for you to soak in and recycle.

Avail yourself of in-store fashion shows. They're often advertised in national fashion magazines if you live in or near a big city. Get on mailing lists of departments where you shop. You may see clothes on bodies that don't look like yours, but you'll walk away inspired—perhaps by how the designer did something new with proportions by mixing up lengths of skirts and jackets in a new and intriguing way.

Look at the newest line of clothing with your wallet in the car. Just enjoy seeing how the designer put pieces together. Maybe she's mixing patterns, textures, fabrics. A store won't carry the whole line (except at designer trunk shows), so ask to see the Look Book, the book that shows that whole line. See how they mixed up the clothes.

Look for role models.

My mother still inspires me with the way she accessorizes everything. A sales associate at Saks Fifth Avenue, intimate with her forties, she fiercely takes "sophisticated eclectic" to glorious new heights. A colleague of mine always looks terrific, and when I bump into her, I check out what she's done this time—paired a classic, full-cuffed trouser with a cashmere V-neck sweater, tying a print neckerchief at her neck, and wearing up-to-the-minute glasses frames.

Although I don't have sisters, I've run into many women whose sisters lead the way. Joan's sister, Diane, took her by the hand and made a fun day out of joint makeovers at the Nordstrom cosmetic counter, a region of the world that Joan would never have dared go to without the support of her sis.

I know I'm not the only one whose teenaged daughters have strong opinions (I don't necessarily share) about clothes.

They're at the peak of their fashion and beauty product years and may be very helpful, or if not helpful, they may at least be patient. Let them take you under their wing. Although they may not understand mature clothing, they have a passion for clothes and being around that can be refreshing, inspiring, and invigorating.

If you're still feeling clueless, rent *Clueless*, the modern remake of Jane Austen's book, *Emma*. The cast of spoiled Beverly Hills high school characters have made fashion a science, and their flair and enthusiasm will delight even the most hardened forty-year-old fashion prude.

What to Do
When Current
Fashion Sucks

*Now and then, at the sight of my name on
a visiting card, or of my face photographed
in a group among other faces, or when I
see a letter addressed in my hand, or
catch the sound of my own voice, I grow shy in the
presence of a mysterious Person who is myself, is known
by my name, and who apparently does exist. Can it be
possible that I am as real as anyone?* ~LOGAN PEARSALL SMITH, *TRIVIA*

IT HAPPENS. The latest fashion magazines arrive, you page
through them, and yikes! Tim Burton's horror creatures, which
used to be confined to the movies, have now taken over the
fashion world. Tree branches are woven into models' hair, war
paint covers their faces, bodies are ensconced in chain mail.
The clothes look ill-fitted on models who look like space trav-
elers. They're never going to snuggle up to your skin. What do
you do when current fashion sucks?

Is this the perfect time to throw your arms up in the air and
confirm the evidence that the world of beauty has passed you
by? Nobody understands you anymore, you might as well be

put out to pasture, and if this is all there is, who cares anyway? You'd rather give up. Well, you're not going to go there.

You're going to remember who you are. You are glorious — a woman of great style, carriage, and confidence. If there isn't inspiration in fashion magazines, your next stop could be catalogs that tend to show more clothes and less art direction. Get on the mailing lists of major department stores. Maybe your friends have some catalogs they're happy with. Ask around. Without the war paint, blurred images, and offensive backdrops, you may see clothes as they actually appear, maybe even on models closer to your age than the nineteen-year-old toothpick models.

If you still aren't inspired, you may need to go directly to the source of beauty and creativity. Head for the hills. Get out for a walk in nature. Go around neighborhoods where people have planted flowers, grasses, bushes, trees. *Go on a beauty walk; take a beauty walking meditation.* Observe the shades of red on a pomegranate tree that hangs over a fence. Notice the reds of the fruit against fall's warm, golden yellow thinning-out leaves. Or take in the stark white birch trees against the brilliant crispness of the cold blue winter sky. Check out the textures of a cactus garden or the various shades of green that clutch close together in clumps of grasses growing next to a creekbed.

Fill your being with what pleases you. Study what makes you happy. Is it the contrast of brightly colored leaves against supporting neutral branches? Is it the cool, matte finish of a large flat stone? What do you see in nature this year that gladdens you? After nature's given you a refresher course in finding beauty, take what you've learned home to your closet. Be adventurous. Mix those greens. Contrast red with a golden yellow. Wear subtle textures of the gray together. Create your own attitude.

The thing to remember about fashion is that it passes. This is comforting. A banquet is presented every season. And then the dishes are cleared away and a new one appears the next season. The seasons run generally like this: Resort wear shows up in November. Spring comes into the stores starting in February. Summer clothes appear in April/May. Fall styles start up in July, and winter is delivered to the stores in September. Like weather, fashion is always changing. There will be something else under the sun next month. The color palettes will change. If what's in the stores now doesn't ring your bells, sit tight. Go play. If you love neutral colors and everything is fluorescent, remember, it'll pass, just like a strong cold front. Fluorescent will leave and something will take its place in a few weeks.

If the clothes are goofy looking and you don't want to deal with them this season, focus on smaller details. Paint your toenails in

a new color. Shop for a new tote bag. Buy a "twin" set—a new belt and a pair of earrings that relates to and harmonizes with the belt. Zero in on a pair of shoes that thrill you. You won't be buying the tops and bottoms this season, but you'll look up-to-date anyway with your well-chosen delightful accessories that make everything look refreshed, like a new coat of paint in the living room.

When the season's clothes don't do it for you, outerwear can. This is the time to buy a great coat or jacket. A super outer piece instantly updates your wardrobe. Or look to innerwear. Buy that underwear you've been dreaming about. **Look good from the inside out.**

Maybe you've been wanting a wooden-handled umbrella, or a new wallet. Put your buying on ice except for these little things that make all the difference. You look at a wallet a zillion times a week, the same with a coat or an umbrella. Direct your thoughts into these crevices. Give the credit cards a rest. Save up. Next season may be your winner, when the silhouettes are perfect on your body, the colors make you twinkle, the fabrics are as comfortable as skin. Enjoy this little respite. Life changes. Just like fashion. Your turn is coming.

Do Something Different

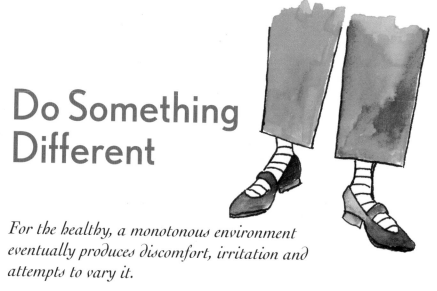

For the healthy, a monotonous environment eventually produces discomfort, irritation and attempts to vary it.

~ SUSANNA MILLER, *THE PSYCHOLOGY OF PLAY*

35

IF YOU'VE BEEN DRESSING YOURSELF for forty-plus years, it's possible you may have gotten into a rut and stayed there. It may look like a clothing rut, but it could be a mental rut. Uprooting a mental rut can do a lot for your wardrobe. How about this one? #1 Bummer Rut: focusing on what's not working rather than what is and staying stuck there. It's easy to say, "What does it matter anymore? I don't have the same body; I don't look as good in clothes anymore. Why bother?" Maybe you had a more up and down figure in your early twenties, and now you have a woman's body, curvy, maybe voluptuous. Fabulous! Your new body expresses more qualities of your womanhood. More sensuality, sexuality, loveliness.

Why do we try to stick to the same-o, same-o, anyway?

Because we're afraid of change? Change is inevitable. We can't keep the sun from rising, we can't keep the weather patterns from heading our way, we can't keep our children from growing up, and we can't keep ourselves from getting older, getting better, changing. It's fascinating how most people find change confrontive. We put off action and use a great deal of energy fighting change, leaving the "problem" to loom bigger and bigger.

Take the plunge. See what's possible when you confront your rut. Instead of putting it off, make a date with yourself to walk into the hip eyeglass store and shop for new frames. Consult with a colorist about your hair. **Be brave**. Call an image consultant for help.

When you embrace change,
solutions are right there at the ready.
They will revitalize you beyond your dreams.

Think about your ruts. You've got two or three. Let me take a guess. Is one of them that your wardrobe has been reduced to a sea of black? Black, black, and more black. How about having clothes for work but having only dregs for your weekend fun wardrobe?

If you're living in black, consider adding color in baby steps—a watermelon T-shirt, a lime green scarf, or a blush-pink beaded, sleeveless, sparkly shell that will transform plain black into just plain gorgeous. Consider a black substitute like midnight navy, charcoal gray, or deep eggplant, which will keep you in the same ballpark as black but will be an energetic change.

Have you been living with rules that you can hardly

remember the source of? Maybe you're the one who never wore black in her life and was told it wasn't your color. This may be your rut antidote—to wear black, at least on the bottom, in a skirt or pant, shoes, and hose. Why not start something brand new? It's fun!

Do you live in sweats? Can't get out of them? Command yourself! Look at current weekend wear and see whether you can't come up with a new uniform that links comfort with style plus a little sex appeal. Come on, we're all sick of seeing you in those ratty sweats. Strut your sweet self into something new for that leisure part of your life.

Always in pants? Play with skirts. Try all the lengths in the stores and see if you come up with something new. Can't get out of jeans? Try a slim pant with a touch of Lycra in it. You'll feel comfortable but different, a good different.

If I haven't named your personal ruts yet, be sure that you do. Once you call them by name, inspired actions will move you out of your ruts and into the light.

Don't go to sleep. When you buy socks, don't go on automatic, looking for what you had before. Take a minute to check out all the possibilities. Don't just buy socks, buy *great* socks. Indulge in patterns and textures that will make looking down at the gap between your pants and shoes a thrill you'll look forward to.

Look through magazines for appealing color combinations and duplicate what thrills you. Try chartreuse and teal, apricot and camel with red-brown shoes and belt, cocoa brown and plum, shades of neutrals together—cement, biscuit, eggshell white.

Wear one color, but play with textures. See how many different textures you can wear in the same outfit. Wear an ivory cashmere sweater set with ivory silk satin flowy pants. Add a chiffon scarf with embossed ivory roses on it. Make it dressy with satin pumps edged in lace, in *ivory*. Wear a moonstone ring, carry a crocheted handbag.

The blessings of age are time and experi ence, love and wisdom and letting go. Practice this in your wardrobe and divine pleasures await you. Who knows? It could lead to a new career, a new relationship, a whole new life.

Get a Tune-up Twice a Year

I have heard with admiring submission the experience of the lady who declared that the sense of being perfectly well dressed gives a feeling of inward tranquility which religion is powerless to bestow.

~RALPH WALDO EMERSON, "SOCIAL AIMS"

I WAS IN THE CAR with one of my teenagers. We were waiting for a woman in a crosswalk when my daughter exclaimed, "Boy, she sure got stuck in the '80s. How can someone get stuck in a decade and not leave it?" she asked in disbelief. The famous Michael Bolton hair, long in the back, short at the top and sides, blond and frizzed, tight acid-wash jeans—yeah, she'd been left behind, that's true. It's probably more glaring to a teenager where a decade claims more than half her lifetime. But it is common. A decade can go by, and a woman may not have changed a thing about her appearance.

Some things are meant to be changed regularly—batteries, light bulbs, oil in the car. Otherwise stuff breaks down and won't work anymore. Other things in your life need changing more often than you think—like hairstyles, makeup colors and application techniques, shoe styles, jewelry styles—or you look broken down. Bring yourself into the current decade. You'll be taken seriously and look bright, as if you've been participating in life and haven't been locked up somewhere for ten or twenty years.

I suggest you plan tune-ups twice a year. Start by going back and doing your homework again. Repeat the Moving Away From/Moving Toward exercise. And do the magazine pulls twice a year too. When you look through your fashion portfolio each spring/summer and fall/winter season, toss out anything that doesn't ring your love bell anymore and add new pictures of current loves. If you're thinking, "Aw shucks, things are going pretty well, maybe I'll skip over this," think again. Ask yourself, *now?* what wants to be expressed Listen closely. You are an evolving human being. You can't stop at a certain year and not move forward. Keep asking yourself the questions that bring you into the present. Review and update what you want from your clothes and your appearance the same way you update your personal or professional goals. Give yourself the opportunity and the pleasure of checking in with yourself and getting the current report on how you want to express yourself. It's a necessity for good health! A little adjustment feels great. Each season you're looking at yourself through a camera lens and bringing yourself more and more into focus.

Plan ahead for this design and listening session. Check your calendar and book time to do the exercises and to look through magazines. Coordinate it to the change of seasons, between winter and spring and between summer and fall. You'll be in sync with the fashion season so if you're getting out there to shop, the clothes will be awaiting you.

Some things creep into life that force fashion updates, like dressing for your high school reunion, attending a professional convention, or going to a wedding—maybe yours! All of these events motivate you to pay attention to yourself, having your hair, nails, and makeup done—much like your in-laws coming in from Chicago somehow motivates you to paint the bathrooms and recycle the last three months of newspapers. Build in your tune-up even if you don't have the pressures of special events.

As part of your twice a year tune-up, weed out your closet when you're changing from winter to spring/summer or summer to fall/winter. Get rid of items that were clearly mistakes or pieces that won't survive another season. Take an hour or so and try on the clothes you're pulling out of boxes or other closets and putting into your current season closet. Do they still excite you? Do they need alterations to fit the current you? Last year's jacket that you lived in might look and feel tired when you put it on this year. Bless it, thank it for its good service, and create a plan for its replacement. Is there a color you're absolutely hungry for this season? If you've changed your hair color, your wardrobe will need some new colors too.

Make an appointment with a freelance makeup artist, someone who is knowledgeable about skin that's been around longer than sixteen years. He or she can update you on colors each season, turn you on to new tools and techniques. If you've been hanging onto your lipstick color for as long as you've been hanging onto those raggedy jeans, you need an update!

Seek out an image consultant. He or she hasn't been living in your routines or ruts, and can hold the vision of your new reinvented self while you're making the changes. An image consultant can educate you about your proportions, new fabrics, and current trends and styles that will work for you. This education pays for itself. They are happily keeping up with everything and are trained to listen to you, to translate your needs into solutions, and to adjust your wardrobe to your life changes. It takes only a few bad purchases to pay for the services of a professional. Contact the Association of Image Consultants International (1-800-383-8831) for a referral.

The scary thing about being in your forties is that you've had a lot of time to unknowingly be doing yourself a disservice. A professional image consultant can get you out of your mistakes or ruts and into clothes and makeup that make you feel terrific. That's worth a few hundred dollars, plus you can say good-bye to those guilt-producing mistakes that took up residence in your closet like bad tenants.

Tricks of the Trade

Time is a dressmaker specializing in alterations.

~FAITH BALDWIN, *FACE TOWARD THE SPRING*

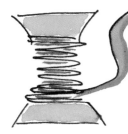

37

I'M AROUND CLOTHES and people's experiences with them on a full-time basis. Here's a collection of tips that have been tested on others and are guaranteed to save you time, money, and heartache.

Give any garment an instant face-lift by going down to your best button store and buying some great, classy buttons. If you're all thumbs with a needle and thread, take them to your dry cleaners and have them make the switcheroo. This one trick will add a perceived $200 value to the appearance of your moderately-priced suit. Clothing manufacturers look for ways to cut corners and one surefire way is to use cheap plastic buttons.

Items essential to a season are the first to fly out the door and unless you think ahead, they aren't going to be there when you need them the most. In fall, stores are full of wool socks, flannel jammies, and long underwear. You may be enjoying the warmth of an Indian summer when you should be looking into the future where cold weather is approaching. When the temperatures dip, you might look in your sock drawer and find nothing. That could be what you find at the stores as well. Don't forget about those hard-working inside garments too — the camisoles, T-shirts, and thin sweaters that you wear with your pants and skirts, whether casual or dressy. Consider buying these crucial items in multiples.

My clients appreciate shopping where there's a long grace period for returns. Creating a wardrobe for a whole season could take a few weeks. As you assemble the likely candidates, put your purchases on a credit card, put the receipt in your wallet, then take your packages home and allow yourself some time to test things out. Give yourself the leisure of planning. You want to see how these potential purchases will fit into your overall plan at home while in front of your own full-length mirror. It's remarkable how different something can look away from the dressing room glare, cluster of sales associates, and pressure of a sale. You'll know what begs to stay and what wants to go back to the store — well within your grace period.

If you don't have that full-length mirror I just mentioned, invest in one now, this week. It's a must. You have to see yourself head-to-toe in order to enjoy the full masterpiece that you are. Hang the mirror in good lighting close to your dressing area.

To protect your pedicure in the summer while wearing closed toe shoes with no socks, take a scissor to your panty hose (hopefully ones that are already trashed) and cut across the foot so you create a little "ped" like you wear when you try on shoes. Also sprinkle foot powder generously into the bottoms of your shoes so your feet don't stick inside your shoes. Foot powder keeps your feet nice and cool.

Speaking of cool, here's what to do to keep from looking drenched in hot weather. Wear a sports bra under a buttoned blazer to help you stay moisture-free. If it's a real problem, apply antiperspirant under your breasts.

Keep a brown and a black magic marker in your closet to touch-up shoes that get scuffed around the outside rim.

Use fabric softener sheets to rub on clothes or hair to get rid of static electricity. If you're traveling, carry baby wipes for instant stain removal.

Use a handsome silver, gold, or fabric eyeglass case as an evening bag when in a pinch. They're perfect for placing on the table in a restaurant or at a dinner party. They'll hold a room key, lipstick, and money comfortably.

A cashmere cape should hit your wish list. You can wear it over casual wear (at a football game), over business suits, or over evening wear where wraps are often a problem. It's also useful to carry when traveling where it makes a cozy airplane or airport blanket.

Do not blindly follow one designer. Become aware of what works for you. If you buy a name brand thinking you'll always look great in that line, you could really miss the mark.

Designers get it wrong too, putting stiff fabrics on curvy silhouettes, for instance. We are such a label-conscious country. Put knowledge before label.

And remember, just because it's

"in,"

doesn't mean

you should be in it.

Hair Dos and Hair Don'ts

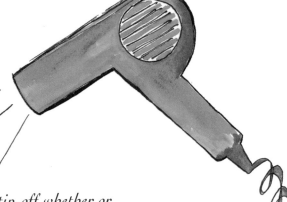

Hair style is the final tip-off whether or not a woman really knows herself.

~HUBERT DE GIVENCHY, *VOGUE* (JULY 1985)

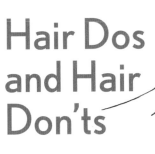

38 GETTING A GREAT CUT or changing to a terrific color can do more to lift your spirits than six months of therapy. It can take years off your face, make you look refreshed, get people wondering if you're having an affair.

A bad cut, or worse yet, no cut at all, going au natural with no shape to your locks, can put you in a bad mood for a long time. You deserve to walk out the door each morning having a good hair day. Here are some dos and don'ts that will help you achieve that.

Go to a new hair designer looking your best self. Introduce yourself to the hairdresser fully clothed the first time, before they get you into a smock. Let the hairdresser see who you are. Here's a place where first impressions will really help to ensure that you get the cut that works with your lifestyle and taste. If you walk in with Ferragamo pumps on your feet and wearing a smart tailored suit, chances are you won't walk out with spiky hair. They don't need to guess as much about who you are if that's clear in the first place. And if you come in, ad executive that you are, in a sleek short black leather skirt and hot pink cashmere sweater set with gargantuan shoes, you probably won't walk out with a pageboy where every strand is in place. Now if you walk in wearing a sweatsuit and no makeup, God help you. Come on! Give these people a break! Give them something to work with. Don't leave them guessing.

Do consider getting your hair cut in a salon where the music is loud, the stylists are wearing clothes from another planet, and the art on the wall is scary. They're up on the latest, and you want the latest information.

If you're letting your hair go gray, and you're darn proud of it, get it cut in a smart, edgy, modern do to keep you looking vibrant.

Find out about the latest techniques. Your frosting could be out, except on birthday cakes, whereas weaving highlights or lowlights is in. There's a big difference. Hair dyed too dark is mercilessly harsh on the skin—unforgiving, brutal. Don't do it. All the lines on your face, even if they're faint, will now stand out like a lit neon sign. Plus, it just looks weird. It's a big announcement—hey, everybody, I dyed my hair.

Loyalty is admirable but detrimental when it comes to hair. You can get lazy, and unless your hairdresser is creative and staying interested in hair developments, attending conferences, and egging you on to try something new, then he or she could be getting lazy along with you and doing the same old thing every month, year after year. Take a risk, get uncomfortable, step out of your rut. Force yourself to consider going to someone new who will have a fresh view of your hair.

Take responsibility for keeping your hairdresser aware of your changes. If he's seen the housewife you for twelve years, show him the leopard-print velvet-pants you, the reckless whimsical you that you've become. Keep your hairdresser up-to-date so he or she can move along with you. If your hairdresser doesn't get it, move on.

If you're new to an area, be on the lookout for those women who have hair similar to yours in texture, weight, color, or body. If you like their cut, then someone is doing a good job. Ask them who it is.

Recognize that someone talented at cutting may not be talented with color. Split the services up between two pros.

Do not be suspicious when a hairdresser recommends a product that they sell at their salon. They aren't making big profits off your $10 shampoo, believe me. Products are always being developed to meet needs. Your hair may benefit from the use of a volumizer, a defrizzer, a mousse, or a gel. Your hairdresser will know what's best.

So what if you bought something last month for your hair that didn't work? Get over it. Be open. Sometimes it takes several tries to get it right. You often buy a few pairs of jeans before you land on the one that really works for you. That's a bigger investment than a $9 hair product. Throw out anything at home that doesn't work anymore or take it down to a women's abuse center for someone else to use. Don't let having products at home that you aren't using be an excuse for turning down something that would improve your chances for good hair days every day.

Let the experts be the experts. Don't be a big know-it-all. They're the ones doing hair five days a week. And don't be a scaredy pants either. Try new things. Be open to a profound change in style or length. Great hair can be your finest feature. Leave your college-days straight, long hair behind and get a do that speaks to your present life and spirit.

Breaking Mother's Rules

Why not be oneself? That is the whole secret of a successful appearance. If one is a greyhound, why try to look like a Pekingese?

~EDITH SITWELL, *WHY I LOOK AS I DO*

39

PATENT LEATHER COMES OUT at Easter, white gets put away after Labor Day, suede shoes are worn during the winter; Mom said so. She grew up when life had neat compartments. Families had moms and dads. Dad went out and worked every day while Mom stayed home with the kids. Families now have same-sex parents, women climb electric poles to fix downed lines, and girls can wear suede all year long, white in the winter as a fashion statement, and patent leather any old time.

Did your mother say this: If one is great, buy two. It is definitely true of condoms, sometimes true about T-shirts, but not true across the board. It could be that by the time you get around to pulling the duplicate skirt out of your closet, it's not in style anymore. Fashion evolves, just like you do, so don't hedge on the future. Enjoy the present.

Look like a lady. Come on, sometimes you just have to look like a tramp. Show some skin, wear slingbacks, paint those toenails red, climb out on the edge. Don't let work swallow you up. Prepare for fun times by creating a wardrobe for those parts of your life. Don't wait till tomorrow, because tomorrow has a way of never showing up. Do it today. Whether it's a pair of canary yellow Keds for your bare feet or a rumpled straw hat you wear to hang out at an outdoor cafe on Sunday while reading the newspaper, add some fun items to your wardrobe.

Honey, you should wear this (fill in the blank). It would look so good on you. Take this test. Next time you're trying on clothes, come out of the dressing room and look in the mirror. Would your mother approve of what you see? If so, then go back, change clothes, and come out in what you like for yourself. Listen to yourself, not anybody else's version of who they want you to be. Accept input from those you trust, then make your own decisions. Educate yourself so you're not so swayed by other people's opinions.

Save that for good, honey. Don't wear it for everyday. Don't save good clothes for good. Wear them now, every day, for five days in a row. Clothes can be expensive. Remember the cost per wear formula? The more you wear your clothes, the less they cost per wearing, which is where the value lies. With some good planning and finding more functions for them, you can combine some of your clothes in ways that take you from work to evening dates. Besides, it feels good to wear well-made, special clothes. Generously create those opportunities.

Never pay retail. You are worth full price. If you come from generations of people who never paid retail, you might feel like a traitor when buying something that's not on sale or hasn't fallen off a truck. What is the source of that tradition? It may have started out from real or felt scarcity. But is that your current circumstance? When you know what you're doing, you know what you love as well as what you want and need, and there's nothing horrible about going out and buying it, sale or not, because you are going to wear the heck out of those clothes. They will serve you on many levels, from the bare necessity of being dressed to the wonderful expression of personal style and personal respect. Don't forget the value of time and energy in the formula for what works for you. It could be that the added activity of searching for sale clothes is stressful and time consuming and threatens your well-being. Put yourself first, not the family tradition.

Don't talk to strangers. Talk to strangers. When you see something you like, someone who's looking great, tell them. "Excuse me, but I just want to tell you that you look terrific today." It's easy, feels good to do, and will contribute to someone's day. This is also a great way to get leads for yourself. If you see someone's hair that you love, ask them who does it.

Buy beige. It goes with everything. Please. Don't begin a wardrobe project centered around something that may be ho-hum for you. If beige makes you feel like a million bucks, then buy beige. Everyone has their own "beige," and by this I mean that you probably have a handful of colors that really become you. Most likely they relate to your coloring—your hair, skin, or eyes. For one person, it's a burnished olive that makes brunette hair just light up. This could be their beige. And building a wardrobe around a color that looks great because it goes with you is smarter than sticking with the color you were once told to stick with. Some people love having two to four colors in their wardrobe that work together. Others need variety in their life. If you're one of the latter, then beige will never do it. Insist on breaking this rule and having a wardrobe that looks like a freshly opened pack of Crayola crayons. Listen to yourself on this one.

Don't you think you're a little old for that? If you have a body shape that allows you to shop in the junior departments with thirteen-year-olds, you could be wondering if Mom's right about this. Use a discerning eye. I have shopped for fifty-year-olds in the junior department and found great pieces that my clients loved and wore for many seasons. Be selective. If you shop completely from that department, you could look out of step. Generally, prices are lower in the junior department. Teenagers aren't spending the same bucks per item that their moms are. The fabrics could also be less expensive looking (because they are less expensive) and the quality not as great to match the price. If you find items that work for you, check them over. You might want to have seams reinforced or buttons sewed on more securely as insurance.

Now, since Mother wasn't around to tell you this, because it started happening after you'd grown up, I think it's my duty to tell you now. Do not leave the gym in your gym clothes and go do your grocery shopping or your mall shopping. People should have to pay for a show like that. Shoppers don't want to be observing soft porn in public, I don't care how cute your butt is. "Now," as Shirley McClaine said in the movie *Evening Star*, "you go home and you rethink your clothing."

Be Kind

To cultivate kindness is a valuable part of the business of life.

~SAMUEL JOHNSON, QUOTED IN
THE LIFE OF SAMUEL JOHNSON
BY JAMES BOSWELL

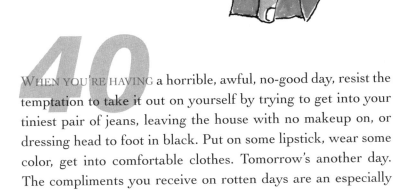

40 WHEN YOU'RE HAVING a horrible, awful, no-good day, resist the temptation to take it out on yourself by trying to get into your tiniest pair of jeans, leaving the house with no makeup on, or dressing head to foot in black. Put on some lipstick, wear some color, get into comfortable clothes. Tomorrow's another day. The compliments you receive on rotten days are an especially sweet-tasting nectar. You deserve it.

I know a woman who was going through a divorce. It was painful and difficult. One day she'd be up and functioning—sort of. The next day she'd take to her bed all day. By the following day, she was strong enough to go out there one more time and tend to the excruciating details of redesigning her life from the basement up. That fall she went to her first back-to-school night as a single, found a lone seat in a sea of doubles, near Sarah's parents, Lindsey's parents, Erica's parents. Walking through the door, she felt that everyone must have been able to see the big empty hole where her guts used to be.

After the class schedules and homework guidelines had been gone over, people got up to leave. As Jennifer's mom, a mom from the old nursery school co-op days, headed toward her, she felt naked and exposed. Jennifer's mom said, "Hi! How are you? You look great! Life's good?"

There was no reason to tell Jennifer's mom the truth. The fact that the summer's events and the separation weren't obvious on the outside was a momentary comfort. Someday she'd be able to say life is good. Receiving the compliment was its own good medicine. She'd catch up with her outer appearance.

Sometimes it feels like your insides are exposed and nothing is protecting you. **But something is protecting you—your clothes**. Clothes that express your taste, highlight your beauty, comfort your body. They precede your words, your thoughts, your fears. They express harmony and balance when you're feeling anything but. They speak before you do. You look "together" even though you're falling apart. **Your clothes can be saying sweet things about you when you can't find a sweet thing anywhere you look**.

All kinds of occurrences can make us grouchy, like divorces, a bounced check, no clean dishes, an empty milk carton, or no messages on the answering machine when we were really hoping for a special one. We get upset for a minute or two, an hour or two, a day or two. What harm is there in letting your clothes, those layers closest to your skin, say nice things about you even while you're grumbling. That's not cheating. Let your clothes light the way, earn a smile, cast a sense of calm, promise poise, excite, scintillate.

I know what I'm talking about. I've heard the testimonials. Mary said, "I feel great since I started paying attention to my clothes. I'm getting so many compliments. This is better than therapy!" Carol said, "I've never felt like such a 'wow.' Even my adult kids are saying nice things to me after years of indifference. It's because my confidence is so high and I feel so good about myself, just as I am."

And I've said it myself. Those months were horrible, going through that divorce. It was me who felt like everyone could see the hole in my gut. But when people's faces brightened and when those who didn't know my pain would look at me and say, "Gee, you look good," it helped me to feel good too. You know what I'm talking about. So instead of it being a once in a while kind of thing, a hit or miss kind of thing, I ask you to stop, appreciate, do all you can to understand yourself and to express yourself in a loving, truthful manner—the you that was designed before you took your first breath, that beautiful, gorgeous you.

And when those compliments come rolling in, don't apologize. Don't bend the ear of the one who complimented you with where you bought it, how on sale it was, how discarded it was, or how insignificant it was. Don't spit on the compliment. Just say, "Thank you." You're precious. Let people tell you that.

Tell yourself that. Be kind. Just this once, and then once more. May the talk that goes on inside your head be inspired by the love of a grandmother's heart. This is the "you" that you have forever. Be kind, sweet, doting, patient, forgiving, curious, and loving. Have fun.

About the Author

Brenda Kinsel has been dressing herself since 1954 when her favorite outfit was the matching Davy Crockett get-up that she and her twin brother wore. She has been dressing others professionally since 1985. Owner of Inside Out, A Style and Wardrobe Consulting Company, she has devoted herself to helping women express themselves through clothing and style, while teaching them how to have a wardrobe that works 100 percent of the time.

A rapt audience of readers in the Bay Area have followed her snappy fashion column in the *Pacific Sun* newspaper. Her essays on clothes have appeared in the *San Francisco Chronicle* and have been part of a charitable event called "Poems & Prose on Sex & Clothes" performed in front of standing-room-only audiences.

Her down-to-earth, humorous approach to fashion earned her fans in radio, and her expert advice has been quoted in *Shape* magazine, the *Los Angeles Times*, the *Cleveland Inquirer.* She was a contributor to the book, *Mastering Your Professional Image, Dressing to Enhance Your Credibility.*

Brenda is a professional member of the Association of Image Consultants International (AICI). She is the current president of the San Francisco Bay Area Chapter as well as frequent workshop leader at AICI conventions.

Ms. Kinsel has led seminars on image, accessories, wardrobe planning, and shopping to audiences at major department stores, professional organizations, corporations, and businesses. Born and raised in North Dakota, she graduated with a degree in education from the University of North Dakota.

About the Designer/Illustrator

Jenny McFee Phillips has been a graphic designer for thirteen years. Her work ranges from developing strategy and launching new products, to creating whimsical illustrations on popular culture.

She is known for her skills in making unfamiliar, difficult subjects intelligible. Her work for organizations has illuminated difficult concepts for a wide audience. Her concepts and designs for cultural institutions in New York and San Francisco have contributed to the increase exposure of a number of arts groups.

Her client list includes Time-Life Books, American Express, The Metropolitan Museum of Art, MTV, Vanity Fair, the American Institute of Architects, GAP Inc., Carnegie Hall, Brooklyn Academy of Music (BAM), NYC Riverside Shakespeare Co., T. Rowe Price, Bechtel, Golden Gate Park and Recreation, and Montgomery Asset Management.

Jenny Phillips is the principal of the newly-formed JuMP Studio in San Francisco. The studio provides art direction, marketing communications, graphic design and illustration.

About the Press

Wildcat Canyon Press publishes books that embrace such subjects as friendship, spirituality, women's issues, and home and family, all with a focus on self-help and personal growth. Great care is taken to create books that inspire reflection and improve the quality of our lives. Our books invite sharing and are frequently given as gifts.

For a catalog of our publications, please write:

Wildcat Canyon Press
2716 Ninth Street
Berkeley, California 94710
Phone: (510) 848-3600
Fax: (510) 848-1326
info@wildcatcanyon.com

More Wildcat Canyon Titles ...

THOSE WHO CAN...TEACH!: CELEBRATING TEACHERS WHO MAKE A DIFFERENCE
A tribute to our nation's teachers!
Lorraine Glennon and Mary Mohler
$12.95 ISBN 1-885171-35-8

A COUPLE OF FRIENDS: THE REMARKABLE FRIENDSHIP BETWEEN STRAIGHT WOMEN AND GAY MEN
What makes the friendships between straight women and gay men so wonderful? Find out in this honest and fascinating book.
Robert H. Hopcke and Laura Rafaty
$14.95 ISBN 1-885171-33-1

STILL FRIENDS: LIVING HAPPILY EVER AFTER (EVEN IF YOUR
MARRIAGE FALLS APART)
True stories of couples who have managed to keep their friendships
intact after splitting up.
Barbara Quick
$12.95 ISBN 1-885171-36-6

girlfriends: INVISIBLE BONDS, ENDURING TIES
Filled with true stories of ordinary women and extraordinary friend-
ships, *girlfriends* has become a gift of love among women everywhere.
Carmen Renee Berry and Tamara Traeder
$13.95 ISBN 1-885171-08-0
Also available: Hardcover gift edition, $20.00 ISBN 1-885171-20-X

girlfriends TALK ABOUT MEN: SHARING SECRETS FOR A GREAT
RELATIONSHIP
This book shares insights from real women in real relationships —
not just from the "experts."
Carmen Renee Berry and Tamara Traeder
$14.95 ISBN 1-885171-21-8

girlfriends FOR LIFE
This follow-up to the best-selling *girlfriends* is a new collection of sto-
ries and anecdotes about the amazing bonds of women's friendships.
Carmen Renee Berry and Tamara Traeder
$13.95 ISBN 1-885171-32-3

AUNTIES: OUR OLDER, COOLER, WISER FRIENDS
An affectionate tribute to the unique and wonderful women we call
"Auntie."
Tamara Traeder and Julienne Bennett
$12.95 ISBN 1-885171-22-6

THE COURAGE TO BE A STEPMOM: FINDING YOUR PLACE WITHOUT
LOSING YOURSELF
Hands-on advice and emotional support for stepmothers.
Sue Patton Thoele
$14.95 ISBN 1-885171-28-5

CELEBRATING FAMILY: OUR LIFELONG BONDS WITH PARENTS AND
SIBLINGS
True stories about how baby boomers have recognized the flaws of
their families and come to love them as they are.
Lisa Braver Moss
$13.95 ISBN 1-885171-30-7

INDEPENDENT WOMEN: CREATING OUR LIVES, LIVING OUR VISIONS
How women value independence and relationships and are redefin-
ing their lives to accommodate both.
Debra Sands Miller
$16.95 ISBN 1-885171-25-0

THE WORRYWART'S COMPANION: TWENTY-ONE WAYS TO SOOTHE
YOURSELF AND WORRY SMART
The perfect gift for anyone who lies awake at night worrying.
Dr. Beverly Potter
$11.95 ISBN 1-885171-15-3

I WAS MY MOTHER'S BRIDESMAID: YOUNG ADULTS TALK ABOUT
THRIVING IN A BLENDED FAMILY
Erica Carlisle and Vanessa Carlisle
The truth about growing up in a blended family.
$13.95 ISBN 1-885171-34-X

Books are available at fine retailers nationwide.

Prices subject to change without notice.